DATE DUE

JUN 0 5 2011		
BYS 7.26.11		
DEC 1 8 2011		
JAN 2 0 2015		
AUG 3 1 2017		

NUTRITION AND FITNESS

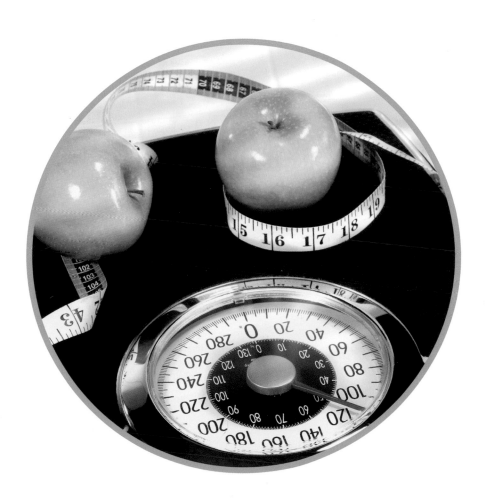

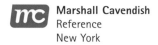 Marshall Cavendish
Reference
New York

Marshall Cavendish

Copyright © 2011 Marshall Cavendish Corporation

Published by Marshall Cavendish Reference
An imprint of Marshall Cavendish Corporation

Website: www.marshallcavendish.us

Library of Congress Cataloging-in-Publication Data
Nutrition and fitness.
    p. cm.
  Includes index.
  ISBN 978-0-7614-7939-0 (alk. paper)
  1. Health--Encyclopedias. 2. Nutrition--Encyclopedias. 3. Physical fitness--Encyclopedias.
  RA776.5.N88 2011
  613.03--dc22

                          2010010235

Printed in Malaysia

14 13 12 11 10   1 2 3 4 5

MARSHALL CAVENDISH
Publisher: Paul Bernabeo
Project Editor: Brian Kinsey
Production Manager: Mike Esposito

THE BROWN REFERENCE GROUP PLC
Managing Editor: Tim Harris
Designer: Lynne Lennon
Picture Researcher: Laila Torsun
Indexer: Ann Barrett
Design Manager: David Poole
Editorial Director: Lindsey Lowe

Other Marshall Cavendish Offices:

Marshall Cavendish International (Asia) Private Limited, 1 New Industrial Road, Singapore 536196 • Marshall Cavendish International (Thailand) Co Ltd. 253 Asoke, 12th Flr, Sukhumvit 21 Road, Klongtoey Nua, Wattana, Bangkok 10110, Thailand • Marshall Cavendish (Malaysia) Sdn Bhd, Times Subang, Lot 46, Subang Hi-Tech Industrial Park, Batu Tiga, 40000 Shah Alam, Selangor Darul Ehsan, Malaysia

Marshall Cavendish is a trademark of Times Publishing Limited

All websites were available and accurate when this book was sent to press.

Key to color coding of the articles

- BODY
- DIET AND NUTRITION
- HUMAN BEHAVIOR
- ILLNESS, INJURY, AND DISORDERS
- PREVENTION AND CURE

Contents

Foreword

It seems as if there is nutrition and physical fitness information everywhere you turn —in magazines, on television, in newspapers, on the Internet, even on billboards advertising full-service health clubs and clinics. Everyone has a new way for you to become healthier! Maintaining your wellness is more than just eating healthier and exercising. It encompasses everything from your body and its parts to your lifestyle choices. With so much advice available, it is hard to know what is reliable and where you can turn for accurate information.

The human body is an amazing machine. When it works well its performance is seamless, and we barely notice that we are functioning. However, when the body does not work well, we become concerned. For example, we barely notice we have a shoulder until it hurts; its presence and function are a normal part of our existence until it ceases to function properly. When there is a problem, we have questions. How to maintain wellness and what the best options are for maintaining health are important issues for everyone to understand.

Modern life has led to new fitness and nutrition challenges. Our relatively sedentary lifestyle and the abundance of junk food, for example, have led to complications such as obesity and its related problems. Strain injuries such as those associated with posture in the workplace have sparked a whole new area of study. In fact, there is probably more research into health issues than anything else. When discomfort or illness strike, we look for answers and may take curative measures before we consult a physician.

With a wide scope of more than 125 articles, *Nutrition and Fitness* provides enough information to answer general questions and can serve as a starting point for more in-depth study. This book captures a diverse assortment of fitness and nutrition topics: acupuncture, the circulatory system, coffee and tea, dieting, exercise, fats, growth, isometric exercises, joints, junk food, massage, pain, physical fitness, reflexes, sports injuries, sunburn, sweat, and yoga, just to name a few. Each article has an easy-to-read layout, and sidebar elements highlight important information for quick reference. As a practical, authoritative resource, this volume is indispensable.

In fact, the ease with which information is available to the reader invites one to continue reading in topic areas that may not be of immediate interest or necessity. Thus, the vital information in this book serves to help the reader proactively address a variety of wellness issues.

Dr. Rashmi Nemade
Rashmi Nemade is a biomedical writer and editor.

Additional related information is available in the 18-volume *Encyclopedia of Health*, fourth edition, and the corresponding online *Health Encyclopedia* database at www.marshallcavendishdigital.com.

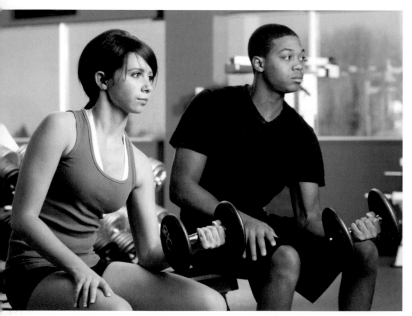

Acupressure

Acupressure is a Chinese healing technique that involves applying pressure to parts of the body to treat disease. One of the concepts of Chinese medicine is chi. This essential life force is said to flow through the body along energy channels called meridians. Specific points, called acupoints, along the meridians regulate the flow of chi through the body. There are hundreds of these acupoints on the human body. When a person is healthy, the flow of chi is in balance with the body and the surroundings. Disease occurs when something upsets the balance among chi, the body, and the environment. Acupressure can then be used to stimulate the acupoints. This pressure unblocks the meridians and restores the flow of chi to treat the disease.

Acupressure is used to treat many medical conditions, which range from allergies and arthritis to migraines and menstrual problems. The treatment may last for several weeks if the problem is acute. Acupressure can also be used as a preventive measure. Regularly stimulating the acupoints relieves daily stresses and strains and keeps the body in balance.

A typical session

Acupressure sessions usually take place in a quiet and relaxed environment. To start, the therapist will ask the patient a few questions and carry out a general medical checkup. The therapist then treats the patient on a massage table or on a mat on the floor. A typical session lasts between 30 minutes and one hour.

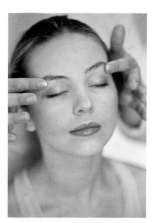

At the end of the session, the therapist may suggest some self-help techniques for the individual to carry out at home.

Acupressure is widely accepted in modern medicine. Some doctors think that the treatment works by stimulating the production of painkilling chemicals called endorphins in the brain. Other doctors think that acupressure stimulates nerve fibers to prevent pain signals from traveling through the body to the brain.

Some therapists believe that using acupressure around the facial area may help reduce wrinkles and improve the appearance of the skin.

SEE ALSO

ACUPUNCTURE • MASSAGE • MUSCLE • NERVOUS SYSTEM • PAIN • REST AND RELAXATION • SKIN • TIREDNESS

Acupuncture

Acupuncture is an ancient healing art that has been used in China for 5,000 years. Now, people in other countries are using this treatment. Acupuncture is based on the belief that energies flow through channels under the skin. When an organ is diseased, the flow of energy is disturbed. Acupuncturists work from a map of the body showing key points along these channels. They believe that they can correct a disturbance by placing very fine needles in the body at one or more points.

Acupuncture certainly seems to help many people, particularly those with arthritis, headaches, digestive problems, asthma, and hypertension. Modern scientists think it either stimulates the body to produce painkilling hormones or triggers pain-blocking mechanisms in the nerve pathways. The treatment is often used to relieve pain and can even be used instead of an anesthetic in some surgical operations and during childbirth. The patient remains conscious but does not experience any pain.

Q & A

I've seen pictures of people with acupuncture needles in them. Is that as painful as it looks?

There may be a slight, brief prick as the needle enters the skin. As the treatment starts to take effect, people usually feel only numbness, or sometimes a slight aching, or tingling.

Do the needles make you bleed?

Usually not, because the smooth, fine, supple acupuncture needles do not damage tissues. Points on the face and ear bleed occasionally because the skin there has a rich blood supply.

How long does it take for the treatment to work?

Acute complaints may improve immediately or within a week or two. Chronic conditions may take perhaps two or three months of weekly treatments, although some benefit should be noticed within a few weeks.

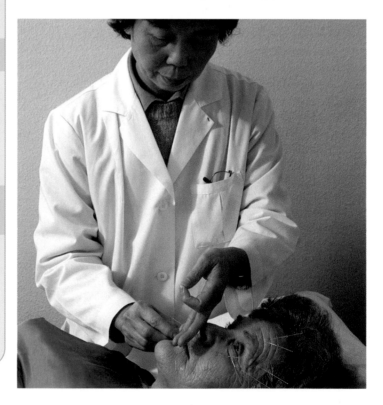

Acupuncture needles have an anesthetic effect powerful enough to allow surgery to take place while the patient is fully conscious. This woman appears perfectly relaxed as needles are inserted in her face.

SEE ALSO

ACUPRESSURE • ANALGESICS • MASSAGE • NERVOUS SYSTEM

Aerobics

An aerobic exercise is one in which the muscles, lungs, and heart work hard enough to make a person feel breathless and sweaty. Many types of exercise, including cycling, brisk walking, jogging, and swimming, are aerobic. This sort of exercise helps people keep fit. Aerobic exercise forms part of an athlete's training, and many people who want to improve their general health go to aerobic exercise or dance classes.

Regular aerobic exercise improves the way the body utilizes oxygen. It increases the amount of air that reaches the lungs, so that more oxygen is carried by the blood to the muscles. It also makes the heart muscle pump the blood around the body more efficiently. Underdeveloped blood vessels are opened, and new capillaries (tiny blood vessels) develop in the muscles.

Aerobic exercise should be performed for about 20 minutes at least three times a week. As people exercise, their fitness increases. This can be shown by recording the heartbeat after the first exercise session; it will be quite fast. As the body becomes more efficient, it will be able to carry out the same program without raising the heartbeat nearly so much. However, people should be careful to build up their exercise program carefully and steadily. They should not tire themselves out by exercising too hard at first. It is best to do about 10 minutes of warm-up exercises before each session and some cool-down exercises afterward.

Aerobic exercise classes are popular and can be helpful, but they should be taught by qualified instructors. People can easily injure themselves if they exercise too hard or in the wrong way.

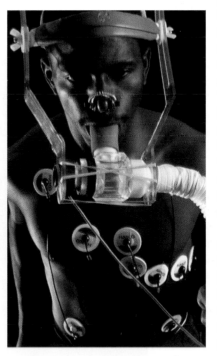

This man is on a treadmill. He is being monitored to find out how much oxygen he takes in during exercise. This test is often carried out to check an athlete's performance during training.

SEE ALSO

EXERCISE • HEART • MUSCLE • OXYGEN • SPORTS INJURIES

Aging

Q & A

My father is a heavy smoker. Will smoking affect his longevity?

Yes, it will. Many people underestimate the risk they are taking by smoking 25 cigarettes a day (even low-tar brands). Smoking will almost always speed the aging process; it can cause death from heart disease and diseases of the lungs and arteries before the age of 60. It affects the skin; people who smoke heavily often wrinkle prematurely. Smoking is not just a minor hazard; it is a major cause of premature death.

My grandmother has shrunk over the past two years. Why?

Height loss is mainly due to thinning of the spinal bones and shrinkage of the disks between the bones. An elderly person's back tends to bow, making him or her bend forward. Maintaining correct posture in earlier life helps to strengthen the back and may reduce later height loss.

A lifetime of healthy exercise has kept this older man fit enough to play competitive tennis. However, it is never too late for elderly people to start improving their fitness levels with gentle activities.

As people grow older, some parts of the body change and become less efficient and even begin to deteriorate. Old skin becomes much less elastic than young skin, for example, and tends to become dry and wrinkled. Hair turns gray, some people's sight may not be good, and many people may become hard of hearing. The heart, bones, and muscles are less strong. Most people even grow smaller as they get older, because the pads between the vertebrae shrink. These changes happen because the body's cells are wearing out and the production of new cells decreases as people get older.

Staying healthy and active

Some people stay young-looking and active far longer than others. This is partly because of the genes that they have inherited. People who come from long-lived families are more likely to live a long time themselves, and some people may also inherit genes for healthy and long-lasting eyes, memory, heart, and so on. However, everyone can increase the chances of a healthy and active old age by keeping fit and healthy when young. Regular exercise as people get older helps keep them fit, supple, and active into old age. Exercise also often improves

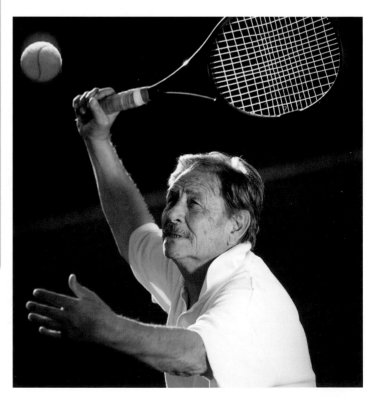

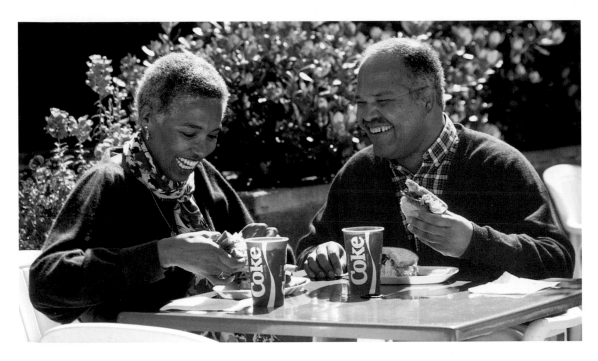

People can have just as much fun when they are old as when they were young. Those who are active and eat a healthy diet can risk an occasional fast-food treat.

the mental attitude toward aging and helps ward off the depression that many older people experience, especially if they live alone. Older people who keep their brains active by reading, studying, and taking an interest in other people and their environment are more likely to stay alert. There are many ways in which elderly people can be encouraged to take an active part in family and community life and to play an important and helpful role. Making elderly people feel useful and wanted is the best way to help them stay young.

Life expectancy

Nearly 12 percent of U.S. citizens are over 65. Because of better health facilities and medical technology, people are living longer than ever before. If a man now lives to 65, he can expect to live another 13 years, and he can expect another nine if he passes the age of 75. A woman of 65 will live 18 more years on average, and a woman of 75 will live 12 more years. By the year 2030, it is estimated that there will be more than 55 million Americans over 65; a great many of them will be women over 85.

SEE ALSO

EXERCISE • HEART • MUSCLE • PHYSICAL FITNESS

Alexander Technique

Q & A

Will the Alexander technique help me lose weight?

No, it is unlikely. However, by improving your posture and learning how to stand upright, you may look taller and give the impression of being slimmer.

Sometimes I get bored, depressed, and tired for no reason. Could the Alexander technique help me?

If you have no specific illness or physical disorder, it may simply be that your system is not working properly; this can lead to low spirits and fatigue. By teaching you to listen to your body and to release any tension you are holding, the Alexander technique can restore your energy levels and general state of well-being.

Do I have to be good at sports to be any good at the Alexander technique?

The Alexander technique is not a physical test; it is a gentle, natural method that works with the body and that can be learned at almost any age, whether you are fit or unfit.

The Alexander technique is not so much a therapy as a process of reeducation. It aims to treat and prevent a wide range of disorders by teaching people to become aware of how they use their body and to make the changes that they find necessary in order to feel some physical or psychological benefit.

The conditions that have been found to respond best to the Alexander technique include back pain, breathing difficulties, neck and joint pain, and stress-related disorders such as headaches and fatigue. It has also been found helpful in such diverse conditions as high blood pressure, spastic colon, asthma, osteoarthritis, and neuralgia.

The Alexander technique is often referred to as posture training but this is not strictly correct, though improved posture does often result from its use. The technique aims to get people to use their body in a relaxed, balanced, and efficient way with natural ease and grace.

Traditionally, the technique is taught on a one-to-one basis and usually requires about 30 lessons at weekly intervals. Each lesson lasts about 30 to 40 minutes, during which time the teacher helps the student look in great detail at the way in which he or she uses the body. Students are taught to look at their personal tension patterns while they are engaged in a range of different activities, which usually include sitting, standing, or walking. They will probably also work lying down on a table. The teacher uses his or her hands, accompanied by verbal instructions, to direct the student to release tension.

How it works

The Alexander technique was developed by an Australian actor, Frederick Matthias Alexander (1869–1955), who believed that "every man, woman, and child holds the possibility of physical perfection; it rests with each of us to attain it by personal understanding and effort." The Alexander technique works on the principle that mind and body form a whole. Although that proposition is now widely accepted, it was considered radical when Alexander came up with his technique at the turn of the twentieth century. The technique does not treat specific conditions, but rather aims to address the source of a problem. In restoring harmony of both mind and body to a person, it is found that many specific problems disappear.

SEE ALSO

ASTHMA • BACKACHE • BLOOD PRESSURE • JOINTS • POSTURE

Amphetamines

Amphetamines are powerful, habit-forming stimulant drugs that are chemically related to the body's own stimulant, adrenaline. Taking amphetamines increases mental alertness and physical stamina, relieves depression, and aids dieting by suppressing the appetite. However, the long-term effects are harmful.

Amphetamines were once widely used until they were found to be habit-forming. People who took them over a period of time needed larger and larger doses to get the effect they wanted. Some people who depended on them became aggressive and violent. Others became listless and depressed. Still other people had mental breakdowns with delusions and hallucinations. As a result, doctors are now understandably extremely wary of prescribing amphetamines. These drugs now have few uses in medicine and are seldom prescribed for any purpose.

Children with attention deficit disorders and hyperactivity are no longer given prescribed amphetamines, although they may be given amphetamine-related stimulant drugs, such as methylphenidate (Ritalin).

Amphetamine abuse

In the 1960s, amphetamine abuse was common. Drugs known as "purple hearts" and "black beauties" were taken by people who wanted a quick high and by students who wanted to stay alert to study for long hours. "Speed freaks" injected themselves with amphetamine solutions. Inhalers containing the drug were available over the counter.

One of the most popular stimulant drugs is the amphetamine derivative ecstasy. The side effects of ecstasy include loss of appetite, irritability, fast talking, abnormal extroverted behavior, fast pulse, heart irregularities, paranoia, hallucinations, depression, bleeding in the brain, and possibly damage to the liver. Extreme and excessive physical activity is commonly brought on by the high produced by ecstasy.

Amphetamine abuse is now less common. People who have become dependent on amphetamines require medical help. They may have a mental breakdown, which results in delusions and hallucinations. Some symptoms of amphetamine abuse are similar to those of schizophrenia, an acute personality disorder that requires hospitalization.

Q & A

I love bicycle racing and want to turn professional in the future. Would taking amphetamines before races improve my stamina?

It is not safe to use these drugs. After several professional cyclists taking part in the Tour de France race died as a result of using amphetamines, national and international sports agencies banned the use of stimulants. If you took amphetamines, you would be not only seriously endangering your health but putting your professional career at risk as well.

My little brother seems to need less sleep than the rest of our family. He's still jumping around at two in the morning. Can my parents just give him some pills to calm him down so we can all get some sleep?

No. Your parents should get some professional advice. Your doctor will advise them whether your brother is really hyperactive or just needs very little sleep. Never give a child pills without medical advice. A dose that has been prescribed for adults will be too strong for a child and will do more harm than good.

SEE ALSO

APPETITE • DIETING • HEART • TIREDNESS • WEIGHT CONTROL

Analgesics

Analgesics are drugs that relieve pain. Some analgesics, including aspirin (acetylsalicylic acid), acetaminophen, and ibuprofen, are mild and can be bought without a prescription. Aspirin and ibuprofen are two examples of a class of painkilling drugs called nonsteroidal anti-inflammatory drugs (NSAIDs).

Aspirin is the most commonly used analgesic drug in the world. It reduces inflammation and fever and is used mostly for minor ailments such as headaches and in the treatment of rheumatic diseases. People may be more likely to survive heart attacks and strokes if they are treated with aspirin and less likely to have those diseases if they take a small daily dose of aspirin.

Aspirin counteracts the effects of prostaglandins (fatty acids, made naturally in the body, that act like hormones). However, large amounts of aspirin can cause intestinal bleeding in adults. A link has also been discovered between aspirin and Reye's syndrome, a rare but very serious condition in children. Aspirin should not be given to children under the age of 12, except with medical supervision. Ibuprofen is a more powerful painkiller and also causes less stomach irritation than aspirin.

Other analgesics have a very strong effect and can be bought only with a doctor's prescription. They include drugs, such as codeine and morphine, that can be habit-forming if taken over a long period.

Q & A

I saw my father drinking an alcoholic beverage even though he is taking an analgesic. Is that a safe thing to do?

If your father is using a mild analgesic such as aspirin, an occasional drink should be safe for him. However, both aspirin and hard liquor can cause bleeding in the gut, so it is wise to avoid the combination. Alcohol should never be taken at the same time as a strong painkiller, because both substances slow breathing and the interaction of the two substances could be dangerous.

I get migraines, but if I don't take a painkiller as soon as an attack starts, the pill doesn't work. Why?

When a migraine attack occurs, the functioning of the intestine, which is controlled by the nervous system, shuts down. Once this happens, there is little chance of a drug's being absorbed in the gut. If you are unable to take a pill as soon as an attack starts, your doctor may prescribe an analgesic in suppository form or an oral drug that will help absorption.

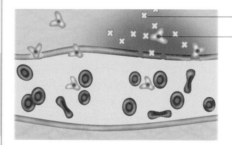

prostaglandin

white blood cell

Prostaglandins cause the blood vessels to widen and leak fluid. White cells move into the tissue, which becomes red and swollen.

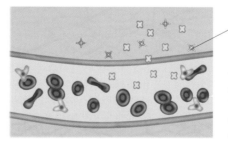

analgesic

NSAIDs limit the release of prostaglandins. The blood vessels return to normal, and swelling and redness decrease.

SEE ALSO

CIRCULATORY SYSTEM • HEART ATTACK • PAIN • STROKE

Anemia

Anemia is a disorder that is caused by an abnormally low level of hemoglobin in the blood. It occurs when the number of red blood cells that contain hemoglobin is low or when the cells contain low levels of hemoglobin.

Hemoglobin picks up oxygen in the lungs and carries it to the body tissues, where it provides energy. If the hemoglobin in the blood falls below normal levels, too little oxygen reaches the tissues. That produces the classic symptoms of anemia: skin pallor, breathlessness, and lack of energy. These symptoms may be accompanied by palpitations (rapid and noticeable heartbeats), fainting, dizziness, and sweating.

Q & A

My mother is pregnant and is getting paler and paler. Could she be anemic?

During pregnancy, the body's demand for essential nutrients, such as iron and folic acid, is increased. The developing fetus depletes the mother's store of nutrients via the placenta, and the mother may then become deficient in one or more of them, causing anemia, unless extra iron and folate are given. Your mother should check with her doctor, who will give her a prescription for supplements if they are necessary.

Types of anemias

A common cause of anemia is a lack of iron, which is an essential component of hemoglobin. Women are particularly likely to experience this deficiency, because of the amount of blood they lose each month in menstruation, especially if they have very heavy periods. Other causes include ulcers that produce slow but steady internal bleeding, cancer of the stomach or intestine, hemorrhoids, and parasites such as hookworms and tapeworms that feed on the blood. Thirst is a symptom of iron-deficiency anemia; anemic children may be irritable and have a tendency to hold their breath.

Without vitamin B_{12} and folic acid, fewer red blood cells can be made, and those that are produced are enlarged. In the United States, people's diets usually contain plenty of B_{12}, but in some people, the stomach lining fails to produce a substance known as intrinsic factor. Without this factor, B_{12} cannot be absorbed, and red blood cell production falls. This condition is known as pernicious anemia. It can cause tingling sensations in the hands and feet, nosebleeds, and, in severe cases, heart failure and nerve damage, as well as the usual symptoms of anemia.

Folic acid deficiency

Folic acid is usually supplied by green vegetables in the diet. A deficiency of folic acid generally occurs in elderly people who are not eating properly, in pregnant women who use extra folic acid to nourish the developing baby, and in people who drink excess amounts of alcohol. These anemias can be treated by increasing supplies of the deficient substance. Iron tablets or shots rectify deficiency anemia in a few weeks. Folic acid deficiency can be treated with tablets and an adequate diet.

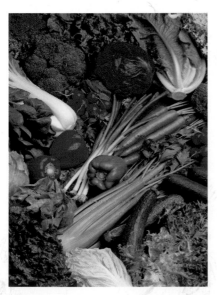

Green leafy vegetables such as salad leaves and spinach are an important source of folic acid and iron, a lack of which can cause anemia.

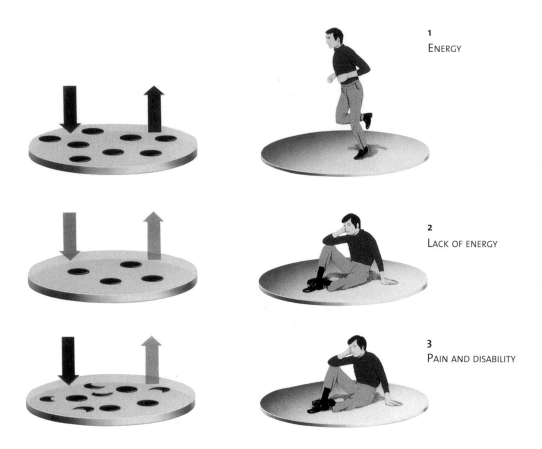

1
ENERGY

2
LACK OF ENERGY

3
PAIN AND DISABILITY

Red blood cells play an important part in anemia. (1) When there are enough chemicals to produce the required number of blood cells, the cells carry adequate oxygen supplies around the body to give energy. (2) When there are not enough chemicals to produce the number of red blood cells required, less oxygen reaches the tissues, resulting in tiredness. (3) Sometimes there are enough chemicals, but a number of red blood cells are malformed. They may block small arteries and cause severe pain and disability.

Vitamin B_{12} and pernicious anemia

If the stomach lining has ceased to produce intrinsic factor, it will never be able to absorb vitamin B_{12}. Regular shots of vitamin B_{12} for the rest of the patient's life will keep pernicious anemia under control, although it will recur if shots are missed.

Hereditary anemias

Sometimes, red blood cells are destroyed more quickly than they can be replaced, causing hemolytic anemia. Two serious types of hemolytic anemias are hereditary. Sickle-cell anemia is present largely in black communities. Thalassemia is present in Mediterranean, Middle Eastern, and Southeast Asian communities. Both types of hereditary anemia are serious and incurable, but they can be helped with blood transfusions.

SEE ALSO

DIET • IRON • OXYGEN • PAIN • VITAMINS

Anorexia and Bulimia

Q & A

My friend has been told she is anorexic but doesn't believe it. Why can't she realize how emaciated she looks?

She is suffering from an abnormal mental state. When she looks in a mirror she sees a distorted body image that initiates, and prolongs, the disease. Your friend should get help from a counselor or doctor.

Sometimes I eat a bag of cookies. Then I'm sorry, so I make myself vomit afterward. Am I suffering from bulimia?

Not unless these binges have become uncontrollable and frequent. Many dieters go on an eating binge after they have been on a strict diet for some time. A binge is not good for the body, but it does no lasting harm. Only when it becomes a way of life should you seek treatment. You seem to feel guilty about overeating, but try to be less emotional about it and attempt to lose weight in a more sensible way.

Anorexia, or anorexia nervosa, is a compulsive desire to lose weight, which goes far beyond any ordinary wish to become thin. Left untreated, it can be fatal. It usually affects young people between the ages of 11 and 30 and occurs more often in girls than in boys. Anorexia nervosa used to be rare, but it is becoming increasingly common, particularly in people from middle-class homes. This is a serious disorder of perception in which the sufferer—a girl, for example—is convinced she is too fat when, in fact, she may be desperately thin. The affected girl may also be frightened of her developing sexuality and feel that if she can keep her childish figure, then she will not have to face up to the problems of adult sexuality. The danger of anorexia must never be underestimated; skilled management by experts is required. Up to 20 percent of cases end fatally.

Some emotionally insecure girls and boys diet drastically to increase their sexual confidence. The idea that being thin is a desirable state is reinforced constantly by television and magazine advertizing that promotes thinness by glamorizing unnaturally thin supermodels.

Addicted to dieting

Normal people who diet drastically can usually stop whenever they choose, perhaps when they have reached their target weight. Their problem is usually to keep to a diet when there is food around them, since hunger is such an unpleasant sensation. Anorexics, once started, cannot go into reverse. They are as addicted to dieting as if they were taking drugs. They may even experience some of the same light-headedness.

Anorexics go to great lengths to hide what they are doing. They may be unusually energetic and insist that they are well. They cook large meals for other people, while eating nothing themselves. They tell lies, saying that they have eaten elsewhere, and become very skilled at hiding food while pretending to eat normally. Some make themselves vomit to get rid of food they have been coaxed to eat, or they use laxatives, diuretics, and even enemas to prevent their bodies from absorbing nourishment. Some anorexics develop a binge-and-vomit pattern called bulimia. They eat large quantities and then make themselves vomit so that they can eat without putting on weight.

Symptoms of anorexia nervosa

The first, obvious symptom of anorexia nervosa is continued loss of weight. It may not be easy for the anorexic's family to recognize the symptom until it has become severe. An unmistakable symptom in a girl is that once her weight has fallen more than around 26 pounds (12 kg) below normal, she stops menstruating. Girls or boys who diet excessively and seem to have a false image of being overweight should be seen by a physician as soon as possible. They may simply need advice and information on the weight they should try to achieve and on a proper diet. However, if they have anorexia nervosa, it is important to begin treatment as soon as possible. The longer the condition goes untreated, the more difficult it is to cure.

Perhaps one in five anorexics eventually dies of starvation or from infections caused by undernourishment. Some become so depressed that they commit suicide. Cures seldom take place without treatment, because victims take pride in their condition. The more distorted their self-image, the more difficult the cure.

Treating anorexia nervosa

The first step is to increase body weight, at least above the danger level. Research indicates that when a patient is below a certain weight, psychotherapy cannot break through the strange mental isolation caused by voluntary starvation. Until a more normal weight is reached, no real communication can take place.

It is usually better to treat anorexics at a hospital. Their food intake must be checked carefully because they tend to hide or throw away food to avoid eating. There is also the possibility that they will fake their weight gain by putting weights in their pockets before they step on scales. This behavior can be monitored more easily in a hospital. Sometimes, patients are made to rest in bed, very often in a room alone, and their food intake is strictly monitored by the nursing staff. In the early phases of treatment, patients may also be given a form of tranquilizer and be fed intravenously. Sometimes, a system of rewards and withdrawal of privileges is used to coax the patient to eat normal food and gain a certain amount of weight.

Once the patient has gained enough weight to be out of danger, psychotherapy can begin. This approach may be required for months or years after the patient is at normal weight. Often, the whole family is given counseling, so that the parents can understand the nature of their child's illness and what causes it.

Bulimia

Bulimia is another eating disorder. It may appear on its own, but it often goes with anorexia nervosa. Its severe form is called bulimia nervosa. This condition is most often present in girls and young women who become convinced that they are overweight, although in most cases, their weight fluctuates between a little above and a little below normal.

EMACIATION AS A SENSE OF ACHIEVEMENT

The longer the illness lasts and the more weight the anorexic loses, the greater is her sense of achievement. She believes that being thin makes her significant and outstanding as an individual. Her behavior focuses attention on herself and sometimes gives her a satisfying form of rebellion against the authority of her parents.

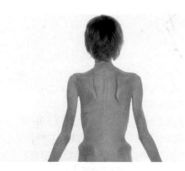
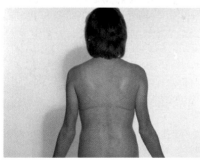

Before and after: This 19-year-old anorexic girl needed hospital treatment. After two months she had a normal body weight.

Many teenagers with anorexia nervosa enjoy cooking for other people, but they are reluctant to eat the food themselves, even if they are hungry.

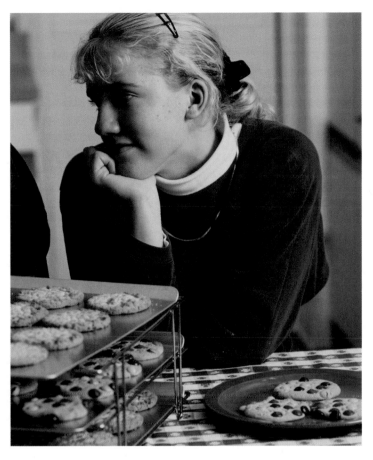

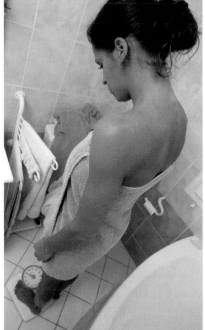

People with anorexia nervosa have an overwhelming desire to lose weight and constantly weigh themselves to ensure that they have not gained any.

People with bulimia eat very large meals, or binge. The fear of becoming overweight then prompts self-induced vomiting. They tend to eat in secret and are unable to control themselves. During binges, they may eat up to 12,000 calories in just a few hours. These binges are often triggered by stress and may take place several times a week or several times a day. The patient may not eat at all between binges. Bulimics do not usually become seriously underweight, as anorexics do, but they can cause themselves physical harm by overloading their systems with food and through the subsequent taking of laxatives. They suffer from weakness and cramps, as well as dehydration, and their teeth may become damaged by gastric acid. Treating their underlying psychological problems often helps the condition.

> **SEE ALSO**
>
> DIET • DIETING • MALNUTRITION • WEIGHT CONTROL

Antioxidants

Antioxidants are substances that mop up some of the harmful by-products of metabolism and prevent the damage caused by outside factors such as cigarette smoke and ultraviolet radiation from the sun.

The body needs oxygen to utilize food in a process called metabolism. Hundreds of thousands of chemical reactions occur during metabolism. Some by-products of these reactions are chemicals called free radicals. Free radicals are also produced when the body is exposed to infections and environmental factors, including ultraviolet radiation from sunlight and pollution such as cigarette smoke. Free radicals attack the cells and tissues of the body and contribute to the effects of aging and major health problems such as cancer and heart disease.

Double defense

The body has two mechanisms to cope with free radicals. The first line of defense involves substances called antioxidants. They destroy free radicals and prevent them from damaging the body. Antioxidants include vitamins C and E and substances called carotenoids (which are present in a wide range of foods) and flavonoids (from sources such as tea and grape skins). The second line of defense involves enzymes that destroy free radicals and repair the damage done to the body's DNA (deoxyribonucleic acid), cell membranes, lipids (fats), and proteins.

Preventing disease

Many medical experts think that by eating more foods rich in antioxidants, such as fresh fruits and vegetables, a person can reduce the risk of certain diseases. Some medical studies have also shown that people can help prevent the onset of certain cancers by taking antioxidant supplements, such as vitamins C and E and carotenoids. The exact benefits of taking these supplements are still uncertain, so most health organizations suggest eating foods that are naturally rich in oxidants. The typical recommendation now is to eat at least five portions of fruit and vegetables every day.

Q & A

When did medical science become aware of free radicals and the role of antioxidants in combating them?

Research began to emerge in the 1970s about free radicals that damage the body's cells and tissues. American chemist and Nobel Prize winner Linus Pauling (1901–1994) proposed that people who took large, regular daily doses of the antioxidant vitamin C had a striking decrease in the number and severity of colds they caught. Many people dismissed his claims, but interest in antioxidants continued to grow.

Antioxidants such as vitamin C, vitamin E, and beta-carotene are present in a wide range of fresh fruits and vegetables.

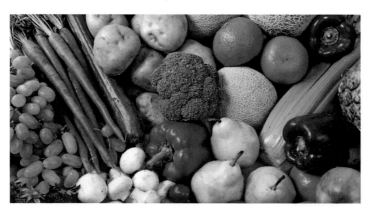

SEE ALSO

BASAL METABOLISM • FOOD AND NUTRITION • VITAMINS

Appetite

Appetite is the desire for food. It is not the same as hunger, which is the need for food. If you want to eat something because it looks and smells good, your appetite is working. When you want to eat something because your stomach feels empty and you feel you really need food, you are hungry.

Appetite regulates how much someone eats and varies greatly from person to person. Some people have a large appetite; they want a great deal of food. Others have a small appetite and eat only a little. The appetite is controlled by an area in the brain called the appestat, which receives signals from the body and tells a person when he or she has had enough to eat. If this system worked perfectly, people would eat just the right amount for the body's needs and no more, ensuring that they had a healthy, balanced diet. However, all sorts of things can affect the appetite. People who are overweight usually eat far more than they need, and underweight people may feel satisfied before they have had enough nourishment. Habit plays a large part. The body can become accustomed to four or only two meals a day rather than three.

When people become ill, they often lose their appetite. However, this may be just the time when they need to eat properly. Pregnant women sometimes have an urge to eat strange things or odd combinations of food, such as pickles and ice cream. Emotional problems and stress can sometimes make people lose their appetite altogether, or might have the opposite effect and make them eat for comfort. As yet, scientists do not really know the reasons why appetite varies so much.

FACTORS AFFECTING APPETITE

Food that looks and smells good tempts the appetite and encourages us to eat more. So does food we know we like. Appetite is also affected by eating habits. People from families who enjoy eating meals together will probably have a larger appetite than those who eat alone. People can train their appetite to some extent by developing sensible eating habits.

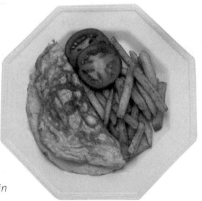
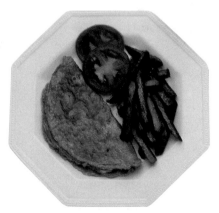

The color of food is important in stimulating appetite. The same omelette and french fries colored blue and green look most unappealing and would probably be eaten only by a person overwhelmed with hunger.

SEE ALSO

DIET • DIETING • FOOD AND NUTRITION • WEIGHT CONTROL

Arthritis

Arthritis is inflammation of the joints. It ranges from brief discomfort to severe, long-lasting pain and serious disablement. Arthritis occurs in people of all ages and can affect one joint or several. In many cases, no one knows for sure what causes arthritis. There are two main kinds of arthritis: osteoarthritis and rheumatoid arthritis.

Osteoarthritis

Osteoarthritis happens as part of the aging process, and almost every adult has some signs of it. It is caused by degeneration of the cartilage, which is the strong, elastic tissue that protects the surface of the joints. The cartilage becomes rough and cracked, compressing the underlying bone and inflaming the tissue lining above it. Osteoarthritis mainly affects the hands and the weight-bearing joints of the hips, knees, and spine. The first symptoms are pain and loss of use of the affected area, followed by stiffness and swelling. In time, the affected joints become distorted. Osteoarthritis gets gradually worse and can be disabling if it occurs in a weight-bearing joint and is severe.

Rheumatoid arthritis

Rheumatoid arthritis is an autoimmune illness in which the body's immune (defense) system works incorrectly, producing antibodies that react against the tissue lining of the joints, causing inflammation, tenderness, pain with movement, and stiffness. This form of arthritis may be triggered by an illness, emotional stress, or shock, which causes a chain of biochemical reactions in the body. Rheumatoid arthritis usually affects adults between the ages of 20 and 55. Rheumatoid arthritis may appear suddenly, starting with a fever or rash, or develop over several weeks. A common symptom is inflammation of the knuckles and toe joints, and the patient may lose weight, become lethargic, and feel generally unwell. The knees, hips, shoulders, wrists, elbows, ankles, and bones of the neck may also be affected. The patient may have great difficulty in moving around and may have to stay in bed. It may be several months before the inflammation dies down, and further attacks can occur. The joints may become deformed and the bones around them weakened.

Still's disease

When rheumatoid arthritis occurs in children, it is known as Still's disease. This condition is fortunately rare. It mainly affects children between the ages of one and three, or between 10 and 15, and the child may have several attacks over the years, ending with the onset of puberty. Each attack may last for several weeks.

Q & A

Is it safe for my father to take a lot of aspirin to ease the pain caused by arthritis?

Yes and no. Because aspirin reduces inflammation and temperature and eases pain, it is often used as a first-line treatment for arthritis. However, when aspirin is taken for a long time, there are two possible side effects: tiny gastric ulcers can bleed or an existing ulcer can flare up.

My grandmother always wears a bandage wound tightly around her arthritic knee. Is this really helpful?

It can be of some help. Bandaging or supporting an acutely inflamed joint can stop jarring movement and, therefore, ease some of the pain. When a joint is swollen, the tissues feel stretched. A support under these circumstances gives a sensation of stability. However, she should always be careful not to make the bandage too tight, because a very tight bandage can reduce the circulation of blood to the lower part of the leg.

The child may have a rash and a temperature that rises from normal in the morning to about 103°F (39.4°C) in the evening; other symptoms can include swollen glands in the neck and armpits, and painful, red eyes. Eye inflammation in Still's disease is serious because it can permanently damage the vision; it requires skilled ophthalmic care.

Other forms of arthritis

Arthritis can be caused by infections, including tuberculosis, rheumatic fever, gonorrhea, and psoriasis. Once the infection is cured, the arthritis disappears. However, it can be triggered at a later date by an injury, such as a blow to a joint. Bacteria in the joint fluid can cause a damaging and dangerous septic form of arthritis. Another type of arthritis that affects the spine and pelvic joints is ankylosing spondylitis.

Many cases of arthritis are treated with drugs such as aspirin and ibuprofen, which help combat inflammation and ease the pain. Steroid drugs such as cortisone can also help the condition but they may have unpleasant side effects. Regular, sensible exercise helps prevent stiffness and loss of movement in the joints and helps muscles keep their strength. Heat treatment can ease painful joints, and swimming in a warm pool is also good exercise for people with arthritis.

A normal knee (below left) compared with an osteoarthritic knee. The smooth cartilage that cushions the joint has degenerated and worn away, leaving the bones to grind against each other. As the bone seeks to heal itself, its surface becomes rough and painful.

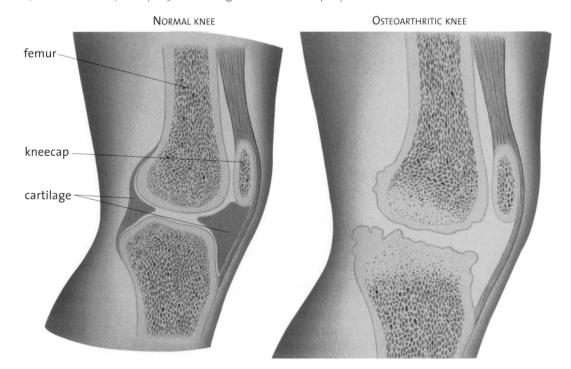

NORMAL KNEE   OSTEOARTHRITIC KNEE

femur

kneecap

cartilage

Relieving the strain of arthritis

Claims are made that special diets ease arthritis, but there is as yet no real proof of this. Too much weight puts unnecessary strain on the joints, so heavy people with arthritis should reduce their weight by eating sensibly and exercising. Operations to replace the hip, the knee, and other joints damaged by arthritis are now common. The damaged joint is replaced by an artificial one made of metal or metal and plastic. This operation is usually successful and gives the patient increased movement and relief from pain. Surgery can also relieve pressure around a joint, can free ligaments that have become stuck together, or can remove inflamed tissue lining a joint if it is greatly affected.

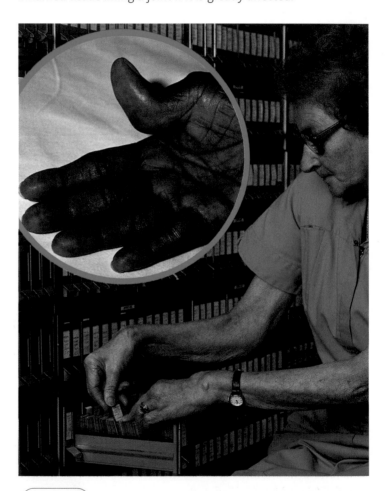

Fine movements with the hands are often difficult and painful for someone suffering from arthritis. People with rheumatoid arthritis need to keep their hands as mobile as possible, but movements may be painful and difficult to make. Sometimes, a joint (inset) becomes so deformed that it cannot be used.

SEE ALSO

AGING • JOINT REPLACEMENT • JOINTS • PAIN • PUBERTY

Asthma

Asthma is a common condition that involves considerable difficulty in breathing. During an attack, asthmatics tend to breathe in with short gasps and force their breath out again with a long wheeze. Asthma is caused by a narrowing of the bronchial tubes when the muscles that line them contract. These tubes lead from the windpipe (trachea) to the lungs.

Asthma attacks are quite common in children, but most people outgrow them in adolescence. Some attacks are mild but others can be extremely bad. Asthma is brought on by a number of different causes, from breathing polluted air to emotional stress. All the different causes of asthma result in the release of one of two chemicals in the body. These chemicals are histamine and acetylcholine, both of which cause the bronchial muscles to contract.

Histamine release is the most common cause of asthma. It is triggered by an allergic reaction to all sorts of substances, including the following: pollen; house dust; certain foods, such as shellfish, eggs, chocolate, and milk; and some preservatives. Sudden strenuous exercise and emotional upsets also cause attacks or make them worse, and the more anxious the patient becomes, the worse the attack gets.

Most asthmatics are prescribed a bronchodilator, which they can use if they have an attack. The bronchodilator contains a substance that opens the bronchial tubes. People with asthma should always carry their inhaler with them, in case they have an attack when they are away from home.

Q & A

What can I do if I forget my inhaler and then suffer an asthma attack?

If you suffer a severe attack, you must go to a doctor or to a hospital emergency room immediately. Otherwise, try to sit still and save your breath.

My father had asthma, and my sister and I now have it. Can asthma run in families?

Asthma does tend to be inherited, especially those types of asthma that are a strong response to an allergy. However, the inherited link is not yet fully understood.

My young brother is asthmatic. Should he play sports?

Yes, all asthmatic children should be encouraged to exercise. Some sports are more likely to cause asthma than others; swimming is the least likely to bring on an attack. Your brother should use his inhaler before taking part.

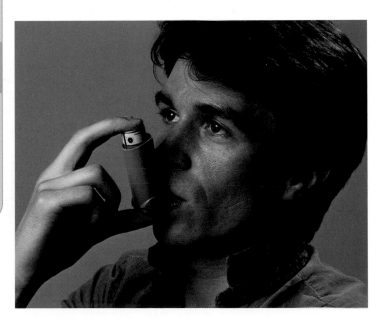

Easy to use and convenient to carry in a pocket, this type of aerosol inhaler relaxes and widens the airways in all but the worst asthma attacks.

PREVENTING ASTHMA ATTACKS

Cause	How to prevent
Infections such as common cold and other viruses, sinusitis, bronchitis	Avoid people with colds, eat a balanced diet, get enough sleep and exercise.
Allergic reaction to pollen, house dust, fungal spores, animal hair	Keep home as dust-free as possible. Do not sit on carpets or rugs. Use foam pillows. Avoid animals. Use air cleaners.
Irritants breathed in, such as gasoline fumes, cigarette smoke, fresh paint, bad odors, cold air	Avoid fumes and smoky atmospheres. Avoid going out in cold air.
Exercise or unusual physical exertion	Avoid strenuous exercise. Use gentle relaxation techniques.
Sudden changes of temperature or air pressure	Avoid sudden temperature changes.
Emotional upset and stress	Identify cause of problem or stress and seek help for it.
Food allergies to milk, eggs, strawberries, fish, tomatoes	Consult allergist to identify allergen and avoid it.
Drug allergies to aspirin, penicillin, vaccines, and anesthetics	Avoid the drugs. A doctor can provide alternatives.

FIRST AID FOR ASTHMA

When a person with asthma has a bad attack, give any drug that the doctor has prescribed and make a note of the exact time. Sit the patient up, leaning slightly forward (resting on the elbows can help). Make sure that he or she can get plenty of fresh air. Give more medication after 30 minutes if the doctor has said that this will be all right. If the attack does not seem to be getting better, telephone the doctor and get ready to take the patient to a hospital if necessary.

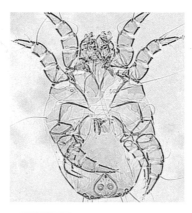

This is a photograph of a house dust mite, viewed from below and magnified many times. These mites are about 0.12 inch (3 mm) long and can be seen only with a magnifying glass. They are found in dust and bedding in even the cleanest home and can trigger an asthma attack.

Treatment of asthma

People with asthma should regularly monitor the state of their bronchial tubes with a peak flow meter, which is prescribed by doctors and is available in large drug stores. This simple device measures the ease with which air can enter and leave the lungs and gives warning of the probability of a dangerous asthma attack. Asthmatics can take inhaled steroids to prevent attacks or help cope with minor ones. These steroids now play an important part in the control of asthma and can reduce the likelihood of permanent lung damage. More severe attacks need prompt treatment from a doctor or sometimes hospitalization. If a severe attack is not treated quickly, the patient may even die. A doctor can inject a drug such as aminophylline, which relaxes the bronchial muscles and takes effect immediately. Hydrocortisone injections also relieve an attack very quickly. Asthmatics should have tests to find the cause of their attacks. Regular, steady exercise, particularly swimming, helps sufferers, but they must be careful not to overdo it. There is no cure for asthma, but current research may lead to one.

SEE ALSO

EXERCISE • HYPERVENTILATION • RESPIRATORY SYSTEM

Athlete's Foot

Athlete's foot is probably the most common foot complaint. It is a fungal infection, like ringworm, that can affect almost everyone, although small children seem immune to it.

The fungus settles in the moist, sweaty areas between the toes, where it lives on dead skin, which the body sheds every day. Athlete's foot may cause inflammation and damage to the living skin. The first signs are irritation and itching between the toes, and then the skin begins to peel. The condition may smell unpleasant. In more severe cases of athlete's foot, painful red cracks appear between the toes and even the toenails can become infected. The nails become either softer or more brittle as the fungus invades the nail substance. In extreme cases, the whole foot swells and blisters.

The fungus that causes athlete's foot can be present on floors and in clothing. People with sweaty feet are particularly likely to develop it. Wearing plastic shoes, which prevent air from circulating around the feet, makes the problem worse. Locker rooms and showers are breeding grounds for the fungus.

Treatment for athlete's foot is simple and soon successful. Antifungal creams should be applied daily while the condition lasts, and for two or three weeks after the symptoms have disappeared, to prevent it from coming back. If the condition does not clear up, the person should see his or her doctor, who may prescribe a drug to take by mouth. To prevent athlete's foot from recurring, the feet, shoes, and socks should be dusted regularly with antifungal powder and the feet should always be washed and dried carefully. Clean cotton or wool socks (not nylon socks) should be worn every day.

Q & A

I have a severe form of athlete's foot that keeps recurring. Will my feet be permanently scarred?

No, because the fungus causing athlete's foot lives only on the superficial layers of the skin, eating dead skin cells.

Can athlete's foot spread to other parts of the body?

The athlete's foot fungus can live on various parts of the body but is not contagious and is unlikely to spread. However, there is a condition similar to athlete's foot that can affect the hands. That should be diagnosed and treated by a doctor.

My sister has athlete's foot. Can she infect the rest of the family?

Not if all family members wash and dry their feet carefully using separate towels and use antifungal powder.

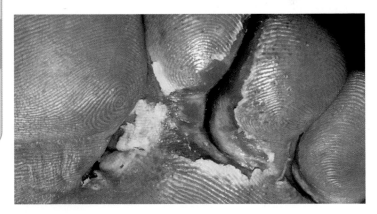

In severe cases of athlete's foot, the skin between the toes becomes painful, red, and cracked. The fungus responsible for the infection grows readily in these warm, moist areas, feeding on dead skin cells.

SEE ALSO

BLISTERS • FEET • PODIATRY • SKIN • SWEAT

Autonomic Nervous System

The autonomic nervous system controls all the body functions that people never really think about, such as heartbeat, food digestion, and breathing in oxygen from the air.

Every day, the body does many things that are taken for granted. Every heartbeat and every breath keeps the body alive, but these events happen automatically, without any thought. The control mechanism for these automatic body processes is the autonomic nervous system.

Inside the nervous system

The nervous system is the body's communication center. Nerve cells are like living electrical switches, which respond to signals from the body's central processing unit—the brain. The brain is a mass of billions of tiny nerve cells. These cells process all the signals from the outside world and decide what to do about them.

The things that people think about, such as opening a door or pressing a button, are processed in "higher" parts of the brain. Things people do not think about, such as blinking and pumping blood around the body, take place in the "lower" parts of the brain and spinal cord, which together are called the autonomic nervous system.

How nerves work

The nervous system works by sending electrical signals down nerve fibers, or axons, from one nerve cell to the next. The axons are the "wiring" through which signals pass along the body, to and from the brain. The nerve cells at the end of the axons transmit or receive the electrical signals. There is a small gap called a synapse between the ending of an axon and the nerve cell itself. Chemicals called neurotransmitters carry the electrical signal across the synapse. The neurotransmitter then stimulates the neighboring nerve cell to produce the electrical signals that pass through the next axon, and so on.

Sympathetic and parasympathetic nerves

In the autonomic nervous system, there are two types of nerves: sympathetic and parasympathetic nerves. Each one uses a different type of neurotransmitter and has a separate effect on the body. For example, parasympathetic nerves in the lungs can make the airways leading to and from the lungs grow narrower. Sympathetic nerves in the same area can make the same airways grow wider. In all cases, parasympathetic nerves are controlled by a neurotransmitter called acetylcholine. Sympathetic nerves are controlled by a neurotransmitter called norepinephrine.

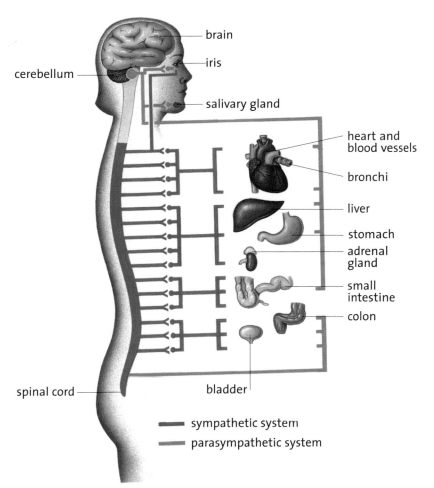

brain

iris

cerebellum

salivary gland

heart and
blood vessels

bronchi

liver

stomach

adrenal
gland

small
intestine

colon

spinal cord

bladder

—— sympathetic system

—— parasympathetic system

*The parasympathetic nervous system,
which is controlled from the brain and
lower spinal cord, interacts with the
sympathetic nervous system, which
is controlled from the spinal cord,
to maintain a balance of the body's
unconscious activities.*

Everyday problems

One minor problem associated with the autonomic nervous system is extremely common—fainting. That occurs when parasympathetic nerves go on overdrive and make many small blood vessels grow wider. The blood pressure then falls and blood flows away from the brain to the body, making the person fall unconscious. To recover from a fainting attack, it is best to lie flat so that the blood flow returns to normal.

Asthma is a much more serious problem. When someone has an asthma attack, parasympathetic nerves leading to the airways in the lungs grow narrower. That makes it very difficult for the person to breathe. Inhaling a drug similar to norepinephrine boosts the sympathetic nervous system, thus widening the airways.

Serious nervous disorders

Many diseases can affect the autonomic nervous system, including AIDS, diabetes, and tumors. Nerve damage can also occur through alcohol and drug abuse. Symptoms of autonomic nerve damage include fainting, fatigue, dizziness, and reduced sweating. Drugs are usually used to control or block nerve pathways leading to the diseased organ. That function copies the effects of natural neurotransmitters. In some cases, surgery is necessary: nerves are cut to relieve symptoms of the condition.

> **SEE ALSO**
> ASTHMA • BLOOD PRESSURE • DIABETES • FAINTING • HEART • NERVOUS SYSTEM • SPINAL CORD • TIREDNESS

Backache

The back is such a complicated structure that it is easily strained or damaged. Backache is one of the most common of all complaints. The flexible spine is normally held in position by the muscles of the back and abdomen. Standing or sitting badly, twisting around, lifting heavy objects, and digging all put strain on the muscles, ligaments, and joints of the back.

Structure of the back

The back runs from the base of the neck to the base of the spine. The spine is a column of small bones called vertebrae. There are 12 thoracic vertebrae at the back of the chest; five much larger vertebrae in the lumbar region (in and below the curvature of the waist); and five fused vertebrae, called the sacrum, that form a triangular bone at the base of the pelvis. At the base of the spine is the coccyx, which consists of three to five small vertebrae. At each end of the spinal column is a ring, or girdle, of bones that provides support for the limbs. At the top of the spinal column, the arms are attached to the pectoral girdle, which consists of the collarbone, the shoulder

Q & A

Will riding my bicycle to school be bad for my back?

No, because on a bicycle your body weight is supported and balanced by the shoulder girdle and the pelvic girdle, with the spine between them. The continual movement of cycling also keeps the back supple and well exercised. However, adjust the handlebars and saddle to suit your height and the proportion of your limbs for comfort and to reduce possible strain on the back.

My sister wears shoes with heels. Will they be bad for her back?

Yes. High-heeled shoes change the body's balance and weight-bearing axis, tilting the lower spine and pushing the weight forward. That puts excessive pressure on the lower part of the lumbar region, causing pain and faster aging of the joints, including the knee joints.

People who have a tendency to backache can help themselves by standing and sitting correctly, with a straight back. A relaxed posture, rather than a stiff, strained position, is ideal.

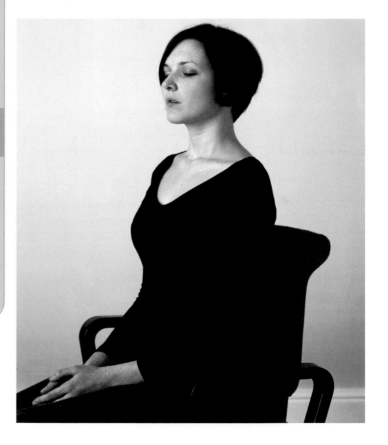

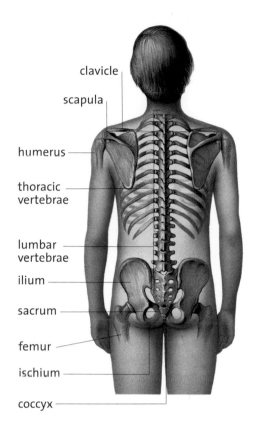

clavicle

scapula

humerus

thoracic vertebrae

lumbar vertebrae

ilium

sacrum

femur

ischium

coccyx

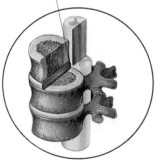

normal disk between lumbar vertebrae

slipped disk pressing on spinal cord

Top: The scapula and clavicle form the pectoral girdle; the ilium and ischium form the pelvic girdle. Bottom: Close-up of vertebral disks in the lumbar region of the back.

blades, and the muscular attachments to the spine. The pelvic girdle at the base of the spinal column is made up of the pubic bones, the iliac bones, and the sacrum.

Types of backaches

Most backaches have no obvious cause. They are the result of some strain that has caused the muscles to go into a spasm. Stress, too, can cause the back muscles to tense and ache. Many people have backaches caused by fibromyalgia, particularly in their shoulders. Fibromyalgia is pain and stiffness in the muscles, particularly those in the neck, shoulders, chest, back, buttocks, and knees. Low back pain (lumbago) is often caused by lifting, twisting, or digging and can come on suddenly or develop over hours or days. It can be so severe that the patient cannot move the back at all. It is probably caused by strained muscles and ligaments and muscle spasm, but it can also be due to intervertebral disk prolapse (slipped disk).

Slipped disks are a very common cause of backache. There is a disk between each pair of vertebrae that prevents friction and eases movement. These disks are prone to wear and tear as time passes, however, and they become thinner.

Osteoporosis, in which the bones become increasingly weak and brittle, can cause the vertebrae to fracture. As a result, older women become shorter as their vertebrae crumble and experience pain as the spinal nerves are compressed.

Ordinary back pain eases in a few days; low back pain may last longer. A doctor may prescribe painkillers and muscle relaxants. A slipped disk may last for a number of weeks, and the doctor may tell the patient to spend a week or two lying flat in bed. Severe cases may be helped by physical therapy or manipulation by an accredited osteopath or licensed chiropractor, who can tell if anything in the back is out of place.

Sleeping on a firm mattress, or with a board under the mattress, gives the back a chance to rest in the correct position.

SEE ALSO

CHIROPRACTIC • MUSCLE • PAIN • POSTURE • SKELETAL SYSTEM • SLIPPED DISK • SPINAL COLUMN

Balance

Balance is the even distribution of weight, allowing one to stand upright and steady. Humans walk on two legs, relying on a highly developed sense of balance to keep them from falling. The body's balancing mechanism is located inside the ears. The ears not only hear sounds but are also responsible for moment-by-moment monitoring of position and movements of the head. If the exact position of the head is monitored correctly, the body can adjust itself to stay balanced.

Balance is a basic skill needed in practically every aspect of life. It is so essential that humans spend their first two to three years of life trying to master balance. It takes another year for children to stand on one leg and even longer to do more balancing exercises, such as walking on a narrow beam. Balance is also critical for any sport, from soccer, tennis, and rock climbing to gymnastics and dance. Being able to sense one's position and balance is the key to being good at sports.

The inner ear

The inner ear tubes that are responsible for balance are well protected by the bones of the skull. Inside the inner ear is a network of tubes filled with fluid at various levels and with

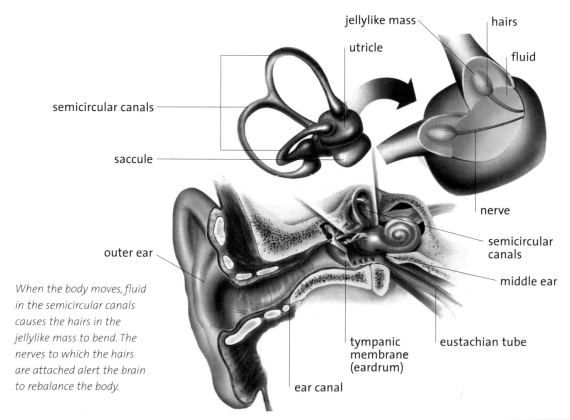

When the body moves, fluid in the semicircular canals causes the hairs in the jellylike mass to bend. The nerves to which the hairs are attached alert the brain to rebalance the body.

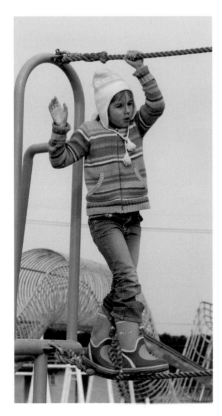

When a child is balancing on a climbing frame, the inner ears are responsible for monitoring the position of the head and body. The ears send messages to the brain to adjust the body's position and keep it upright.

differing angles. The tubes most directly involved in balance are the utricle, the saccule, and the semicircular canals.

The utricle and saccule are involved in detecting the position of the head. Each of these tubes contains a pad of cells with fine hairs called hair cells that are coated with a jellylike fluid. When the body is upright and the head is still, the hairs remain still or unbent, and a resting signal is sent to the brain. If the head turns, the fluid moves inside the tubes, bending the hairs with it in the same direction as the head. Bending the hairs prompts nerve impulses that tell the brain the head is moving. When the head leans forward, backward, or sideways, the hairs bend in different ways. New messages are sent to the brain, telling the muscles of the body to adjust position. If a child starts to run, the hairs are pushed back as though the child were falling backward. The brain receives this information and sends signals to the muscles to make the body lean forward and restore balance.

Above the utricle of the ear are three semicircular canals. At the base of each canal is an oval mass of jelly containing the tips of sensitive hairs. The canals pick up information about when the head starts and stops moving. That is important in quick movements. Unlike the utricle and saccule, the fluid inside the semicircular canals stays still, pushing against the hairs. The hairs send messages to the brain to take action. Sometimes, even when the head stops moving—for example, after someone has been spinning around—the fluid inside the semicircular canals continues to move. That causes dizziness. For instance, when dancers are first learning to pirouette in ballet, they often get dizzy from the continual turning. However, as they practice, their ears and body get used to this motion.

The cerebellum

The part of the brain that is most responsible for directing the action of the muscles in keeping the body balanced is the cerebellum. The cerebellum collects information not only from the balancing organs in the ears, but also from the eyes, neck, spine, arms, and legs. These systems work together to keep a person balanced. For example, when playing tennis, an athlete must keep his or her eyes on the ball and run to keep up with the ball, while keeping the rest of the body ready to respond to the ball's position. All of the body's balancing systems must be used to carry out these actions.

SEE ALSO

BODY SYSTEMS • FAINTING • MUSCLE • SPORTS • TIREDNESS

Basal Metabolism

Metabolism encompasses all the chemical processes in the body that allow a person to grow, survive, and reproduce, using food as fuel. The rate of metabolism varies according to the amount of energy a person expends and from one person to another. The minimum constant rate of metabolism that is measured several hours after eating, when the body is at rest and in a room at normal temperature, is the basal metabolism. That is the energy needed to keep the body running. Metabolism consists of two distinct processes—catabolism and anabolism. Catabolism is the breakdown of complex substances in food into simpler ones, releasing energy in the process. This energy is converted into useful work through muscle activity. A certain amount of energy is lost as heat. In anabolism, food materials are adapted to be stored as energy or used by the body in growth, reproduction, and defense against infection. The term *anabolic* refers to the building up of complex substances from simple substances.

An adult whose food intake is too low uses anabolic food reserves and loses weight. If more food is eaten than is needed, the surplus energy is stored as fat. A person doing a lot of heavy work or strenuous exercise needs more energy, and therefore more food, than a secretary. A child needs more food than that required simply to provide energy, because the surplus is used in growing. People who have a low basal metabolic rate burn their food slowly and have to do extra exercise to avoid putting on weight. People with a high basal metabolic rate are usually able to eat what they like without gaining too much weight.

Q & A

I am no longer losing weight on my diet. Is this connected to my basal metabolism?

Yes. Less food causes the body to lower its basal metabolism in an attempt to slow down and conserve energy. That can cause a plateau effect—no further weight loss can be achieved. A regular routine of cardiovascular exercise helps raise the basal metabolism and thus the rate at which calories are used.

EXPENDING ENERGY

The energy a person expends is measured in kilojoules (kJ); one kilojoule is equivalent to around 4.2 kilocalories (kcal) or big "C" Calories. An average-size man has a basal metabolic rate of around 7,110 kJ a day (1,700 kcal); an average-size woman's rate is around 5,850 kJ a day (1,400 kcal). The rate varies between people.

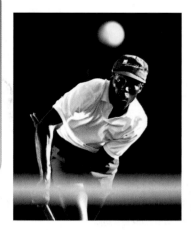 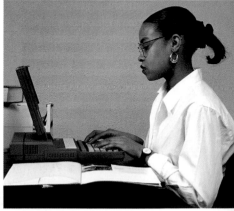

People expend different amounts of energy depending on their activities. An average person burns 1,750 to 2,000 kJ (420–480 kcal) per hour playing tennis (left) and only 300 to 350 kJ (70–80 kcal) sitting at work (right).

SEE ALSO

ANOREXIA AND BULIMIA • CALORIES • DIET • EXERCISE • FOOD AND NUTRITION • OBESITY • WEIGHT CONTROL

Black Eye

A black eye is a dark bruise and swelling around the eye. A black eye normally looks a lot worse than it is. Despite the name, it is not the eye that turns black but the eyelid and skin around the eye. A black eye is caused by a blow to the eye or nose. The eye itself is normally not harmed, because it is protected by a ring of bone and flesh called the eye socket, or orbit.

Under the surface

The scientific name for a black eye is a periorbital hematoma. *Periorbital* means "around the orbit." *Hematoma* is the medical name for bruising and swelling. A bruise is created when the skin is damaged without being cut open. The damage breaks the blood vessels in the skin, and the red blood released beneath the skin gives the skin its dark color. More blood rushes to the area so the body can start to mend the damage. As a result, the bruise fills with liquid and swells.

Thin skin

The eye area bruises more easily than most parts of the body, because the skin is stretched around the eye socket and has only a thin layer of soft tissue beneath. When this area bruises, there is not much room for the blood, so it spreads out below the thin, stretched skin. That is why a blow to the eyebrow or nose can make the whole socket and eyelid look bruised and swollen.

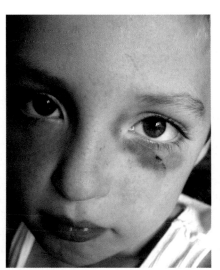

The eyelid might get so swollen that the eye becomes closed. When this happens, it is important to visit the doctor so he or she can check that the eye itself is not damaged.

Holding something cold on the sore eye feels good and makes the blood vessels in the area shrink, which stops blood from getting to the bruised area and reduces the amount of swelling.

SEE ALSO

BRUISES • CIRCULATORY SYSTEM • ICE THERAPY • PAIN • SKIN

Q & A

Why is raw steak the traditional remedy for a black eye?

A clean, raw steak provides moisture, coolness, and softness in a form that will mold itself neatly to the shape of the eye. It has no other beneficial properties and it is an expensive compress. A cloth wrung out in cold or iced water is just as good and readily available at no cost.

The school dance is in five days. How can I disguise a black eye I just got playing basketball? I've already bought my dress!

You could wear sunglasses, but carefully applied makeup should go a long way toward disguising the black eye. Apply foundation in a slightly lighter color than your normal skin tone. Wear eye shadow in a color similar to the bruising. Remember that most black eyes go away in six to eight days, so in five days' time, the color you will have to cover will be much reduced.

A black eye can be very painful but often looks worse than it is. It usually takes around a week for the bruising to heal.

Blisters

Q & A

I have a blister on my heel. Should I pop it?

It is best to leave blisters as long as possible before popping them, because of the risk of infecting the underlying skin. Some blisters will be more comfortable if the fluid is drained with a sterile pin or needle by a doctor, but unless they cause discomfort, blisters are best left alone, covered by a small bandage. Large blisters need medical attention.

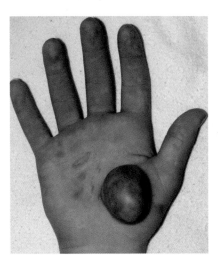

A large and painful blister like this one should be seen by a doctor. There is a high risk of infection if such a blister is popped, because of the large size.

Blisters are swellings caused when fluid collects between the outer and inner layers of the skin. They are caused most often by friction, such as rubbing or chapping. Wearing shoes that do not fit properly and doing heavy work with the hands when they are not used to it are two common causes of blisters. All types of burns, including a bad sunburn, can also raise blisters. The heat and damage to the deep layer of the skin cause an almost immediate outflow of fluid from the blood capillaries; the fluid then lies in the form of blisters under the skin. Sunburn blisters tend to be small and numerous. The skin will start to peel a few days later. Other blisters are caused by bites and stings, illnesses including chicken pox, and infections. Cold sores are made up of a cluster of tiny blisters, caused by a virus called *Herpes simplex*. They sometimes appear on the lips or side of the mouth after a cold. If the cold is severe or the skin is exposed to too much sunlight, the virus will multiply, and crops of blisters will form.

Symptoms and treatment

A common friction blister causes feelings of heat and pain, and by the time these symptoms have been noticed, a blister will have formed. Similarly, a blister arising from a direct burn appears a few minutes after the accident. Blisters from stings and bites appear more slowly and cause itching and a swelling of the surrounding skin. Chicken pox begins as small, dark red pimples, which within a few hours turn into blisters that look like droplets of water. Where there are multiple blisters with no symptoms, the cause is more likely to be eczema.

The common friction blister is rarely dangerous, but in other types of blisters there is a danger of infection. Bacteria can enter the body and breed, forming pustules, which delay healing or spread infection. If large areas of the skin are blistered, there is also a risk that the body will lose a lot of fluid, causing the patient to become seriously ill.

People with large blisters or blisters that appear for no known reason should see a doctor. Other blisters should be kept clean and covered. If the area will get more friction, the blister should be opened with a sterile needle to let out some of the fluid. Otherwise, a blister should be opened only if it is really painful. To treat a friction blister, first cool and clean the area. A small adhesive bandage can be used to cover a small blister.

SEE ALSO

EXERCISE • FEET • PAIN • SKIN • SUNBURN

Blood Pressure

As the heart pumps blood around the body, the pressure of the blood in the arteries varies. Blood pressure is highest when the heart is pumping blood into the arteries (systolic pressure) and lowest when the heart is resting between beats (diastolic pressure). These two pressures are measured together in checking a person's blood pressure.

The "normal" level of blood pressure varies greatly from one person to another and increases as someone gets older. For young and middle-aged adults, a pressure of 120 (systolic) and 80 (diastolic) is considered normal. That is written as 120/80. A blood pressure of 140/90 would be a little worrying; a pressure of 160/90 is definitely high and needs treatment.

Low and high blood pressure

Some people have low blood pressure. That is nothing to worry about, although it can make them feel dizzy, particularly if they stand up suddenly. Blood pressure can fall seriously low with certain infections; when a person loses a lot of blood or is in shock after an accident; or after a heart attack.

High blood pressure, or hypertension, is common in people living in the developed countries of the world and is a serious problem. The increased blood pressure damages the walls of the arteries and can lead to a coronary thrombosis, a heart attack, or a stroke. Arterial damage from high blood pressure can also lead to serious disturbances in the functioning of the brain, eyes, kidneys and other organs, and muscles.

As a precautionary measure, everyone should have his or her blood pressure checked regularly by a doctor.

The pulse

The pulse is the regular throbbing that is made by the heart as it pumps blood through the arteries and around the body. The pulse can be felt in a number of the arteries that lie near the body's surface, including the artery on the inner surface of the wrist. Taking someone's pulse tells a doctor whether the heart is beating regularly and how fast and how strongly it is beating. The pulse also gives information about the condition of the person's arteries. The normal pulse rate is around 70 to 80 beats a minute in an adult. That rate can rise to more than 120 beats a minute with exercise or as the result of a fever.

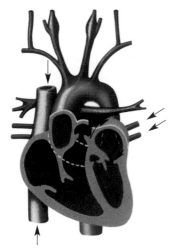

The minimum (diastolic) pressure is taken when the heart has filled with blood from the head, arms, lungs, and body and is fully distended.

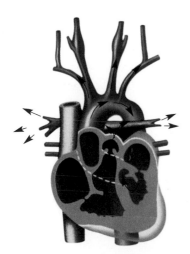

The maximum (systolic) pressure is measured when the heart is pushing the blood out into the body and lungs.

SEE ALSO

CIRCULATORY SYSTEM • HEART • HEART ATTACK • STROKE

Body Systems

The organs of the body are major units such as the heart, lungs, stomach, liver, kidneys, skeleton, and brain. Each organ is made of tissues, which in turn are made of cells. The cells are complex collections of cell organs (organelles) bathed in a chemical-rich fluid. Each cell contains deoxyribonucleic acid (DNA), which incorporates the genes that determine the characteristics, such as skin and eye color, that children inherit from their parents.

There are several main types of tissues, and each organ contains at least one kind of tissue. Epithelial tissues, for example, are sheets of tissues that cover or line the organs of the body. Epithelial tissues include the skin, which covers the outside of the body.

Connective tissues are those that connect or fill out the structures of the body. They include ligaments and tendons.

Skeletal tissues include all the bones of the skeleton and the soft gristle known as cartilage. Muscle tissues enable the body and its component parts to move and work.

Nervous tissue is the communication network of the body, linking all the parts and carrying messages to and from the brain.

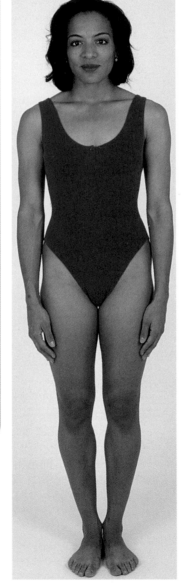

Right: The human body consists of a number of systems, each with its own job to do, yet all working together as a unit.

Far right: Muscle tissue consists of fibers that contract. Epithelial tissue lines and covers the surface of internal organs.

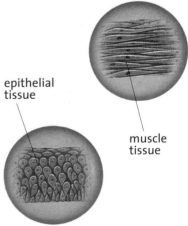

epithelial tissue

muscle tissue

The skeletal system

The skeleton, or skeletal system, is the framework that supports the body. The bones that form the skeleton are linked by flexible joints so that the body can bend and move. The bones are held in place at the joints by bands of tissue called ligaments.

The skeleton is made mostly of bone. While a baby is in the uterus (womb), however, its skeleton is made of a softer, more flexible substance called cartilage. As a child grows, the cartilage is gradually replaced by hard bone. Adults still have cartilage in the lower part of the nose and ears, at the ends of long bones, and between the front ends of the ribs and the breastbone.

The muscles that enable a person to move make up most of the body's flesh. Many muscles, known as skeletal or voluntary muscles, are attached to the bones by cordlike tissues called tendons. These muscles are stimulated by messages from the brain that are carried along the nerves. As a result, muscle movement can be controlled. Other muscles, known as smooth or involuntary muscles, work automatically. They include the muscles of the digestive system and the heart. Heart muscles have the power to contract spontaneously and rhythmically.

The circulatory system

The heart is a pump that drives the blood around the body. Together, the heart and blood make the circulatory system. Blood is used to carry food and oxygen to all the cells of the body and to take away their waste products. The blood flows through a complicated network of tubes, known as the blood vessels, which forms the body's plumbing system. This pipeline system of vessels is extremely long; in a full-grown man, it can total more than 60,000 miles (97,000 km). The system carries about 10 pints (4.7 l) of blood. The blood picks up oxygen from the lungs and is then pumped through the biggest blood vessels, known as the arteries, to all parts of the body. The arteries divide into smaller blood vessels, called arterioles. From there, the blood flows through fine tubes called capillaries to all the body's tissues. The capillaries distribute oxygen and other nutrients to the tissues and collect waste products. The blood then flows back to the heart through a series of medium-size tubes, known as the veins. Blood is returned to the lungs, where it gets rid of carbon dioxide and picks up fresh oxygen.

The immune system

All around are bacteria and viruses that can make people ill. The body's immune system helps protect people against disease. The first barrier in the immune system is provided by the skin.

Skin is a kind of epithelial tissue that covers the surface of the body. The surface that can be seen is made of dead cells (1). Below is living tissue containing nerve cells (2), sweat glands (3), hair follicles (4), fat cells (5), and blood vessels (6).

Below left: The skeleton is made of hard, living bone tissue. The bones are hinged at joints. The knee joint allows up-and-down, but not sideways, movement. The ball-and-socket hip joint allows the thigh bone to rotate. The joints between the bones of the toes are highly flexible.

Below middle: The power to move the bones is provided by muscles. A single muscle acts not alone, but with one or more other muscles. When a muscle contracts, it pulls on a bone; its opposing muscle relaxes to let the bone move.

Below right: Blood supply is vital to bones, muscles, and all the other tissues. Blood flows through blood vessels, carrying food and oxygen to the cells and waste materials away from them.

However, germs can enter through wounds or be injected by insects such as mosquitoes. Germs can also enter the lungs through breathing if they are not trapped and expelled in the mucous lining of the respiratory system. Once inside the body, germs encounter white cells in the blood, which attack and kill them with the aid of antibodies. If germs are swallowed, acids in the digestive system help destroy them. If the immune system breaks down, the consequences are serious.

The respiratory system

The organs of the respiratory system consist of the mouth and nose, trachea (windpipe), and lungs. Just as the heart is a pump for the blood, the muscles between the ribs and the diaphragm act as pumps for air, contracting to increase the volume of the chest so that air is drawn into the lungs. Like the heart, this mechanism works automatically, pulling in fresh air, rich in oxygen, and expelling waste air that contains carbon dioxide. Unlike the heart, the lungs are not completely automatic.

Oxygen absorbed from the air is used by the body to convert food into energy. The converted food is carried to the cells by the

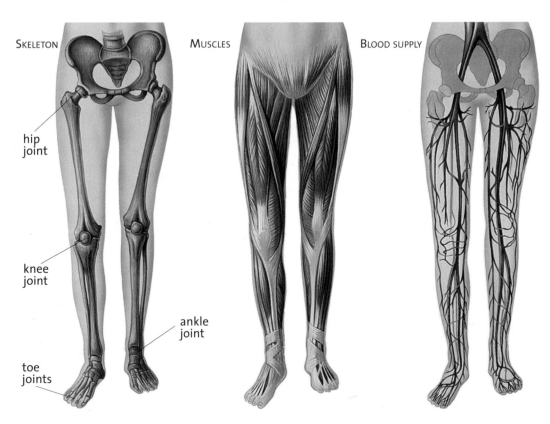

SKELETON   MUSCLES   BLOOD SUPPLY

hip joint

knee joint

ankle joint

toe joints

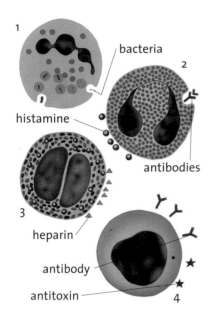

A variety of white blood cells performing their various jobs: swallowing bacteria (1); reacting to antibodies and histamine (2); releasing heparin to stop blood from clotting (3); and releasing antitoxin to neutralize antibodies (4).

blood. In the cells, waste carbon dioxide gas is picked up by the blood and returned to the heart. It is then pumped to the lungs and expelled from the body. This process is called respiration.

Breathing is known as external respiration. Air is drawn in through the nose and filtered to get rid of harmful substances such as dust and bacteria. As air goes down through the trachea to the lungs, it is warmed and moistened.

The trachea divides into two smaller pipes called bronchi, located inside the lungs. In turn, the bronchi split into a network of smaller tubes called bronchioles. The bronchioles branch into tiny sacs, called alveoli, where oxygen is delivered to the blood and carbon dioxide is returned.

The digestive system

Food and drink are the body's fuels and the raw materials from which the body can replace or repair worn-out and damaged cells. Before the blood can take these supplies to the cells, they must be broken down into a form in which they can be used. This process is called digestion. Digestion begins in the mouth when the food is chewed to break it into small pieces before swallowing. The saliva in the mouth is the first of many powerful substances that act on the food. From the mouth, the food passes down a long tube, called the esophagus, to the stomach. Muscles in the stomach wall knead the food to soften it further, and chemicals called gastric juices act by breaking down proteins.

The respiratory system consists of the nose (1), mouth (2), trachea, or windpipe (3), and lungs (4). During breathing, most of the work is done by the diaphragm (5), a large sheet of muscle that lies below the lungs. The lungs are protected by the rib cage (6).

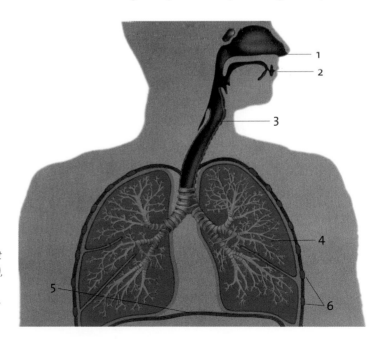

From the stomach, the partly digested, semiliquid food passes into the intestines. First, it enters the small intestine, a coiled tube around 20 feet (6 m) long, where the food is finally broken down into the form of fats, amino acids, and glucose. In this state, the food is absorbed into the bloodstream through tiny projections, called villi, on the walls of the small intestine.

From the small intestine, what remains of the food passes into the large intestine. Most of the useful substances have by now been absorbed into the blood. The remainder is waste, including roughage, such as vegetable fibers and seeds, living and dead bacteria, dead cells from the walls of the upper part of the digestive system, waste gastric juices, and water. As this waste material passes through the large intestine, most of the water is removed, and the solid waste is eventually expelled from the body through the rectum and anus in the form of feces.

The urinary system

Waste substances that have been broken down in the body are carried by the blood to the kidneys. They remove waste materials and surplus water from the blood, producing a liquid known as urine. Urine then passes, via the ureters, into the bladder, where it is stored. Once there is a sufficient buildup of urine in the bladder, the body is stimulated to excrete it via the urethra.

The glandular system

The glands are the body's factories, making substances that the body needs and processing waste products. There are two kinds of glands: exocrine and endocrine. Exocrine glands secrete their products into ducts, or channels, that carry them inside or outside the body. Exocrine glands include the liver, tear ducts, salivary and digestive glands, and mammary glands (which produce milk). Endocrine glands are ductless; they secrete hormones straight into the blood. They include the pituitary gland, thyroid gland, and adrenal glands. These hormones control growth, reproduction, the rate at which food is burned, the level of blood sugar, and the body's emergency response to fear and stress. Hormones can also be released by other organs, such as the brain, the kidneys, and the placenta, or fetal life-support system, in a pregnant woman.

The nervous system and senses

The nervous system is the control mechanism for the body. Its central switchboard is the central nervous system (CNS), which comprises the brain and the spinal cord. The central nervous system receives and interprets messages from the rest of the body and sends instructions through nerves to the muscles,

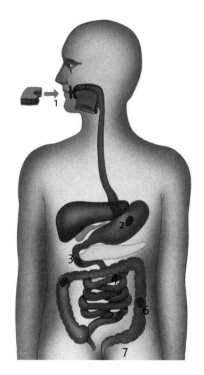

This diagram shows the digestion of a cheese sandwich. Proteins, fats, and carbohydrates are broken down into small molecules and absorbed into the blood to be used by the cells. Digestive juices in the mouth (1) act on the food, which passes into the stomach (2) and on to the duodenum, the first part of the small intestine (3), and the jejunum (4) and ileim (5). The broken-down food passes through the intestine walls. Waste matter enters the large intestine (6), where water passes into the blood. Finally, waste passes through the rectum (7), which is the end of the intestine, and out of the body.

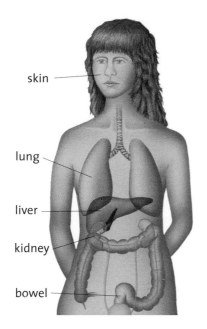

skin

lung

liver

kidney

bowel

organs, and glands. The nerves are like telegraph wires, along which the electrical messages travel to and from the body's senses. The senses link the brain with the world outside the body.

Humans are sensitive to sights, sounds, tastes, smells, touch, heat, cold, hunger, thirst, tiredness, and pain. The eyes are the organs of sight. The ears hear sounds and help people maintain their balance. Taste and smell are linked to the digestive system. Aromas trigger the saliva needed for digestion. People's senses tell them when the body needs to have food or rest, when it needs to avoid danger, or when there is a malfunction or pain.

The reproductive systems

A man's and woman's reproductive organs enable a male sperm to fertilize a female egg to produce a baby. Women have ovaries, which produce ova (egg cells). Once a month, one or more ova pass down the fallopian tubes to the uterus, where the egg can be fertilized. Men have testes, glands that produce sperm cells.

Above: The body removes waste through the skin (water and salt), lungs (carbon dioxide), liver and gallbladder (bile), kidneys (urea), and bowel (feces).

Right: Glands regulate metabolism, aid digestion, produce sweat, and control growth and reproduction.

Far right: The central nervous system consists of the brain and spinal cord, from which pairs of nerves radiate all over the body to form the peripheral nervous system.

Below: The female reproductive system consists of the ovaries, fallopian tubes, uterus (womb), and vagina.

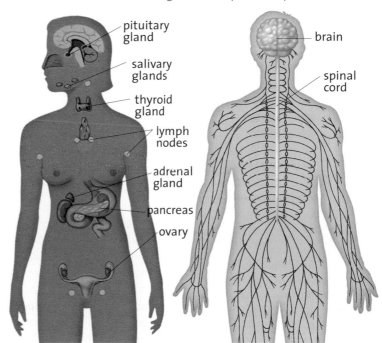

pituitary gland

salivary glands

thyroid gland

lymph nodes

adrenal gland

pancreas

ovary

brain

spinal cord

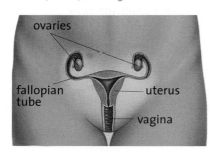

ovaries

fallopian tube

uterus

vagina

SEE ALSO

AUTONOMIC NERVOUS SYSTEM • CIRCULATORY SYSTEM • DIGESTIVE SYSTEM • GLANDS • HEART • LIGAMENTS • MUSCLE • NERVOUS SYSTEM • RESPIRATORY SYSTEM • SKELETAL SYSTEM • SKIN • TENDON

Bruises

A bruise is a patch of dark or discolored skin that can occur on any part of the body. It is caused by a bump or blow that damages the small blood vessels (capillaries) within the lining of the skin. Blood oozes out of the capillaries, giving the skin the familiar dark red color of a bruise. The area swells as serum (watery fluid) from the blood collects there. The platelets in the blood start the clotting process, which limits the area of the bruise and plugs the leaking blood vessels.

A bruise takes about three to six days to heal. During this time, the body reabsorbs the blood, and the bruise fades to bluish purple, greenish blue, and then yellow, before fading away completely. Small bruises are best left to heal on their own. Pressing gently on the bruise with a cloth soaked in cold water or with an ice pack limits the pain and swelling.

Complications

A bruise under a toenail or fingernail should always be shown to a doctor, because the tiny bone beneath the bruised nail may be broken. The doctor may decide to release the blood from under the nail to relieve pain and reduce the risk of infection. That helps stop the whole nail from turning black. Very large and swollen bruises should also be seen by a doctor.

When bruises occur with open wounds or lie over bony structures such as the skull and ribs, they may hide a fracture. In the case of bruises to the face and scalp especially, it is always advisable to see a doctor to rule out any underlying fracture or other damage to these areas.

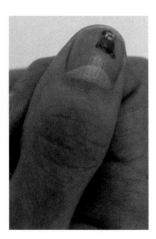

Some people bruise more easily than others. Children, for example, often have many bruises, usually because they are likely to have many minor falls and bumps. Elderly people also bruise easily, because their skin is less elastic and their capillaries become increasingly fragile with age.

Anyone who seems to bruise very easily and with little apparent cause should be checked by a doctor to eliminate other problems.

SEE ALSO

BLACK EYE • CIRCULATORY SYTEM • FRACTURES AND DISLOCATIONS • ICE THERAPY • SKIN

Q & A

I bruised my shin really badly while playing football. Is it possible that I have damaged the bone in some way?

Although the shinbone (tibia) is very near the surface of the skin, it is strong and does not fracture easily. Nevertheless, you should see a doctor if you are worried.

I have noticed that my bruises often take longer to fade than other people's bruises do. What is the reason for that?

Several factors could be adding to the delay. Your body's clearing mechanism may be slow in reaching the affected area, or the bruising may be extensive and so may take longer to clear anyway. Alternatively, if a hematoma (a localized collection of blood) occurs, you may need medical help. Finally, there is a slight possibility that you may have a deficiency either of vitamin C or of blood platelets, which will slow down the clotting process. You should see your doctor.

A bruised fingernail may cover a small broken bone, so medical advice should be sought if a nail is injured.

Calcium

Calcium is a mineral. Together with the mineral phosphate, it is the basic constituent of bones and teeth, and it gives them their strength. Calcium has other important functions in the body. It is essential for muscle contraction and for the transmission of nerve impulses from nerve endings to muscle fibers. Calcium also helps blood to clot and is required for cell functioning.

The body absorbs calcium from food. During digestion, calcium passes through the intestines into the blood. Excess calcium is excreted in the urine. The remainder is stored in the bones and teeth or reabsorbed into the bloodstream. Parathyroid glands in the neck produce parathyroid hormone and control calcium levels. If calcium levels are low, parathyroid hormone acts on the bones and teeth to release more calcium and to reduce loss in the urine. If calcium levels are too high, less parathyroid hormone is produced.

Milk, cheese, eggs, fish, and meat are the richest sources of calcium and should be included as part of a balanced diet.

Q & A

Is it dangerous to eat too much calcium in my food?

No. The body regulates how much calcium it requires and absorbs the correct amount from your blood. Excess calcium is passed out in the urine. However, taking too many vitamin D pills can upset the balance. If the absorption system goes wrong, kidney stones can result. A low-calcium diet helps avoid this.

My grandmother, who is in her sixties, recently broke her arm. Is it possible that her bones have weakened as she's grown older?

Yes. The estrogen present in women before menopause helps build up calcium in the bones. After menopause, osteoporosis (thinning of the bones) may develop. Your grandmother must have an adequate diet. Extra calcium and biphosphonate drugs will also improve her condition.

People need calcium throughout life to keep their bones and teeth healthy. The main dietary sources of calcium include milk, cheese, eggs, meat, fish, and leafy green vegetables.

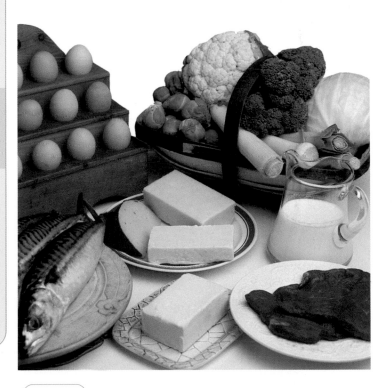

SEE ALSO

DIET • DIETING • FOOD AND NUTRITION • GLANDS • MINERALS • VITAMINS

Calories

The body needs energy for all its activities—sitting, running, breathing, and digesting. People get this energy from the food they eat. The energy value of food is measured in kilocalories. One kilocalorie is equivalent to the amount of heat needed to raise the temperature of one kilogram of water by one degree Celsius.

The number of kilocalories that people need depends on how much energy they use. An active person such as a coal miner, construction worker, or athlete needs more kilocalories than someone who sits at a desk all day, such as a student, doctor, or office worker. Drivers also need fewer calories.

Energy needs also vary according to age, sex, body size, climate, and health. It has been estimated that about 2,000 kilocalories per day are needed to keep the body functioning normally. For example, a woman needs between 2,100 and 2,400 kilocalories per day; a man needs between 2,700 and 3,200 kilocalories per day. However, these figures are an average guide only; they will vary with the age and weight of the individual concerned and with the amount of exercise taken outside work.

Protein, carbohydrates, and fat all provide energy. Proteins and carbohydrates yield around 4 kilocalories per gram; fats yield around 9 kilocalories per gram. Kilocalorie intake also determines weight. If a person consumes more kilocalories than needed, the excess is stored as fat.

Q & A

Which exercise is best for burning calories?

It depends on what exercise you prefer and how much time you have. For example, burning off an apple (about 100 calories) would take 20 minutes of walking, 12 minutes of bike riding, 9 minutes of swimming, or 5 minutes of running. Burning off a hamburger (about 350 calories) would take 67 minutes of walking, 43 minutes of bike riding, 30 minutes of swimming, or 18 minutes of running. By counting calories, you will have a better idea of how to adjust your exercise schedule.

CALORIES USED IN EVERYDAY ACTIVITIES

Activity	Calories used per hour
Sleeping	65
Sitting	75
Standing	110
Typing	140
Walking slowly	200
Running	400
Swimming	500
Walking upstairs	1,100

SOME CALORIFIC VALUES

Type of food	Calories per 100 g	% Water content	% Protein content	% Fat content	% Carb. content
Beefsteak	250	56.9	20.4	20.3	0.0
Brown rice	100	11.7	6.2	1.0	86.5
Butter	700	13.9	0.4	85.1	a trace
Cabbage (boiled)	15	95.7	1.3	a trace	1.1
Cheese	400	37.0	25.4	34.5	a trace
Fish (cod)	100	65.0	20.5	8.3	3.6
Oranges	70	64.8	0.6	a trace	6.4
Potatoes (boiled)	100	180.0	2.5	a trace	15.9
Sugar (white)	395	a trace	a trace	0.0	99.9
Walnuts	350	5.0	15.0	64.4	15.6
White bread	200	38.2	7.8	1.3	52.7
Whole milk	65	87.0	3.4	3.7	4.8
Whole wheat flour	340	15.0	13.5	2.5	69.0

SEE ALSO

CARBOHYDRATES • DIET • FATS • PROTEIN • WEIGHT CONTROL

Carbohydrates

Q & A

Why does eating a lot of carbohydrates make me gain weight but eating a lot of proteins doesn't?

The human body uses proteins and carbohydrates in different ways. Carbohydrates are used for energy; when they are not being used, they are stored by the body as fat. Proteins are used to make structural tissue (muscle, bone, skin), enzymes, some hormones, and neurotransmitters. Therefore, proteins are not stored by the body as fat.

Because she gains weight when she eats carbohydrates and fats, my friend claims that the two things have the same caloric value. Is that true?

No. There are three basic food groups: carbohydrates, proteins, and fats. Carbohydrates and proteins contain roughly four calories per gram; fats contain nine calories per gram.

French fries and an apple are both rich in carbohydrates. The apple is better, healthier and less fattening, not because of the starch in the potatoes but because of the fat used for frying them.

Food consists of three main groups: proteins, fats, and carbohydrates. Carbohydrates are the main source of energy for the body because they provide the fuel, glucose, on which all cells depend. These cells play a vital role in the proper functioning of the internal organs and the nervous system and in heart and muscle contraction. Carbohydrates are made by plants in a process called photosynthesis. Humans get this type of food from certain plants or from animals that feed on plants.

There are two main types of carbohydrates: starch and sugar. Most carbohydrates eaten are starches, the stored food in plant seeds. Starch is made of complex chains of molecules linked with units of glucose. Starch is indigestible unless it is cooked. It is present in grains, vegetables, and fruits. Grains include whole-grain bread, rice, oatmeal, cereals, pasta, tortillas, and crackers. Sugars, including glucose, galactose, fructose, sucrose, and lactose, are present in all sweet foods, such as cakes, cookies, candies, and honey, and in sweet drinks. During digestion, enzymes in saliva and the intestines break down carbohydrates into simple sugars such as glucose, which are absorbed into the bloodstream. Some glucose is transported to the liver, changed into a form of starch called glycogen, and stored. As the body uses glucose, the stored glycogen is changed back into glucose and released into the body to provide energy. This process is controlled by hormones, particularly insulin from the pancreas.

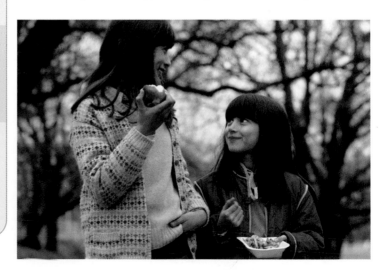

SEE ALSO

APPETITE • CALORIES • DIABETES • DIET • DIETING • FATS • FOOD AND NUTRITION • PROTEIN • SUGARS

45

Celiac Disease

Celiac disease is a particular condition in which food, especially fats, cannot be properly absorbed. Celiac disease is a genetic disorder in which there is a sensitivity to gluten, the insoluble protein present in wheat and other grains, which causes the stickiness in dough. Gluten is a mixture of two proteins: gliadin (which causes the problem) and glutenin. In people with this genetic mutation, the immune system is sensitive to gliadin, treating it as a foreign substance and developing antibodies to it, which attack the intestinal lining.

For digested food to be absorbed, a large surface area is needed. Although the small intestine is about 20 feet (6 m) long, its internal surface would not provide nearly enough area if it were plain and smooth. To aid absorption, the surface area is increased by millions of tiny, fingerlike protrusions called villi. Molecules of digested food pass through these villi to get into the bloodstream, before being carried to other parts of the body.

In celiac disease, the antibodies that attack the intestine have their most obvious effect on the villi, which become stunted and almost flat. The diagnosis can be positively confirmed by performing a biopsy. The patient swallows a small, spring-loaded device (Crosby capsule), which is attached to a tube. When it is triggered, a sample of intestinal lining is retrieved through the tube. Microscopic examination reveals the defects in the villi.

Q & A

My brother has celiac disease. Am I likely to develop it as well?

Celiac disease does run in families, though just how it is passed on is not clear, and not everybody with celiac disease has relatives who suffer from it. There is a controversial theory that celiac disease can be brought on by feeding infants foods containing gluten at too early an age, before their immune system can cope with foreign proteins. So it may be due to a combination of hereditary and dietary factors.

Symptoms and treatment

Celiac disease causes weight loss, diarrhea, abdominal pain, anemia, bloating, distension, and bulky and fatty stools. There may also be bone softening from mineral and vitamin deficiency. These symptoms are due to food retention in the intestine and nutritional losses from failure of absorption. Treatment involves excluding gluten from the diet. That is difficult, because gluten is used widely in foods such as bread, cakes, soups, sauces, hot dogs, and even ice cream. Expert advice is necessary. Extra vitamins and minerals may be required.

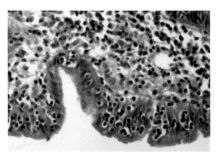

The above biopsy shows normal villi, the projections that line the small intestine and absorb nutrients. The stunted villi on the right show celiac disease.

SEE ALSO

ANEMIA • DIET • DIGESTIVE SYSTEM DISEASES AND DISORDERS

Chiropractic

Chiropractic is a complex and highly specialized manipulative therapy, which aims to correct disorders of the spine, joints, and muscles by the skillful use of the practitioner's hands and without the use of drugs or surgery. It is similar in some ways to osteopathy. Chiropractic restores mobility to the spine and takes pressure off the nervous system, which connects the spine with all the major organs of the body.

Spinal disorders are common and cause problems not only to the spine, but also to other areas such as the arms, hips, legs, and shoulders. They can cause back problems such as sciatica, lumbago, and slipped disk, and are even linked to complaints such as asthma, constipation, digestive troubles, and headaches.

Consultation and treatment

An initial consultation lasts about 30 to 45 minutes, during which the chiropractor takes a detailed case history and discusses the current problem before examining the patient. After taking the pulse, blood pressure, and blood or urine samples, and checking reflexes, the chiropractor examines the spine while the patient sits, stands, walks, and lies down. He or she is able to spot any irregularities in the way the patient uses the spine and thus find out exactly where the spine is malfunctioning. X-rays may be taken, to pinpoint the area of damage and the extent of the problem.

The first treatment usually begins at the second visit. The chiropractor uses special manipulative techniques to restore normal function to the musculoskeletal system, probably with a rapid thrust to the vertebra. The type of technique depends on age, build, and general health. Massage and trigger points are often used to loosen knots and to warm tense, painful muscles. Ice treatments may be used to reduce pain and swelling.

Each manipulation, known as an adjustment, takes seconds, and the patient is asked to breathe deeply. Adjustment is not painful, but there may be a cracking noise, which is often the worst part of the treatment. After treatment, the body may be slightly sore and may need a couple of days to settle down.

The number of sessions needed depends on whether the problem is acute or chronic. Acute problems can be treated relatively quickly, usually with about 10 to 12 treatments over a period of six to eight weeks. Chronic cases take longer.

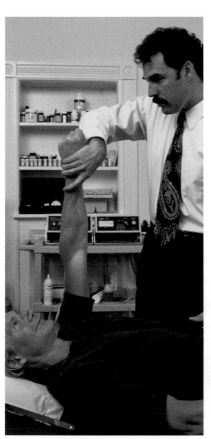

A chiropractor uses manipulation, known as adjustment, on a patient's arm in an attempt to bring the joints and muscles of the body into alignment.

SEE ALSO

BACKACHE • MUSCLE DISEASES AND DISORDERS • OSTEOPATHY

Cholesterol

Cholesterol is a fatty substance that forms part of the wall around the body's cells and is used in the production of some of the body's hormones. Normally, the body produces as much cholesterol as it needs. Cholesterol is also eaten in certain foods.

Eating a great deal of cholesterol may cause high levels of the substance to build up in the bloodstream. That may cause problems. Cholesterol is laid down in the walls of the arteries to cause the condition known as atherosclerosis, leading to hardening of the arteries, coronary artery disease, and strokes.

People at risk

A number of factors contribute to the risk of arterial or heart disease. Smoking and a family history of these conditions are as important as the level of cholesterol in the blood. People in the United States get about 40 percent of their food energy from fats. Surveys of other groups of people who traditionally eat a less fatty diet suggest that if this figure was reduced to below 30 percent, cholesterol levels would probably be lowered. Such a reduction could be achieved by replacing fats with carbohydrates (starchy foods such as bread, potatoes, and rice). Also, fats of animal origin—saturated fats—seem to increase cholesterol levels, whereas unsaturated fats, such as sunflower, safflower, and corn oil, do not.

Although not all scientists agree about the part played by cholesterol in the diet in causing atherosclerosis, it is sensible for people to avoid eating too much food that is high in cholesterol. That includes foodstuffs such as butter, cream, cheese, eggs, and meat. Fish and poultry contain less cholesterol than beef, lamb, and pork. Unsaturated fats from vegetables, such as sunflower oil or olive oil, are healthier than saturated fats from animals. Regular exercise also lessens the risk that cholesterol will build up in the artery walls.

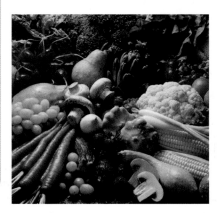

Q & A

Does a high level of blood cholesterol run in families? Several of my relatives have had heart attacks. Is there any connection?

Yes, there are some well-known medical conditions in which abnormalities of the fats and cholesterol in the blood are inherited. People thus affected may need intensive treatment with both diet and drugs.

My brother has always been teased about being fat. Does this mean that he has a high blood cholesterol level?

Not necessarily. People who are very overweight consume more food than they need, storing the excess food energy in the form of fat. Their blood cholesterol, however, depends largely on the makeup of their diet, and your brother may also be eating the wrong kinds of foods. Try to get him to cut out fast food, ice cream, cakes, and candies.

To maintain the right cholesterol level, it is important to eat a varied diet. The foods shown here are a healthy choice.

SEE ALSO

CARBOHYDRATES • DIET • EXERCISE • FATS • HEART • STROKE

Chronic Fatigue Syndrome

Q & A

My brother has been diagnosed with chronic fatigue syndrome. My father thinks he is just lazy. Could my father be right?

Certain psychological states mimic chronic fatigue syndrome (CFS) outwardly, but if a doctor has diagnosed CFS in your brother, his condition will be mainly physical. However, CFS does cause some psychological depression. Support from those near him, such as his family and close friends, will help.

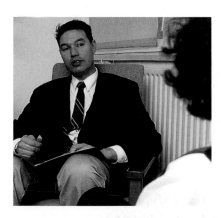

Cognitive behavior therapy has been used to treat chronic fatigue syndrome. During cognitive therapy, the patient is taught to analyze his or her thought processes, to identify negative trains of thought, and to adopt a more positive outlook.

The term *chronic fatigue syndrome* is now most commonly used for a condition that involves severe fatigue and psychological disturbance. The condition can be made worse by exercise. Chronic fatigue syndrome has had many names in the past, including myalgic encephalomyelitis, post-viral fatigue syndrome, epidemic neuromyasthenia, Otago mystery disease, and Icelandic disease. Although detailed clinical investigations into the condition have been carried out, in most cases they have failed to reveal any organic abnormality that could account for the symptoms and the disablement.

Chronic fatigue syndrome is more common in women than in men. The fatigue experienced is not simply muscle fatigue and is quite different from the weakness experienced in disorders such as muscular dystrophy. In chronic fatigue syndrome, there is often a strong psychological element, with the sufferer experiencing mild to severe depression. As a result of the accompanying depression, there has been a degree of skepticism surrounding chronic fatigue syndrome. In part, this is because doctors suspect that the symptoms mask an underlying psychological problem. However, the cause or causes of chronic fatigue syndrome have yet to be identified. Although depression is often present, it has not been established whether depression causes the disorder or arises as a result of the disorder. Other theories link chronic fatigue syndrome with viral infections or suggest that it can arise as the result of a personal trauma, such as a death, separation, or loss of work.

Critical attitudes by doctors and others in the medical field have not been helpful and have caused much distress to sufferers. Although it is important to establish whether or not the condition has a physical cause, it is also vital to acknowledge that people with the symptoms of chronic fatigue syndrome deserve help. Such a persistent disruption of normal living indicates a disorder of the whole person.

Because of the failure to discover an organic cause, doctors have not been sure how to treat the condition. In some cases, antidepressant drugs have been helpful. In others, cognitive behavior therapy has been used. This type of therapy is not concerned with the cause of the condition. Instead, cognitive therapy concentrates on persuading the sufferer to live as normal a life as possible, often with excellent results.

SEE ALSO

EXERCISE • LETHARGY • MUSCLE • TIREDNESS

Circulatory System

The circulatory system is the body's transport system. It carries food, oxygen, water, and other essential materials around the body to nourish and repair the cells; waste products are carried away and expelled from the body. The circulatory system consists of the blood, the blood vessels (veins, arteries, and capillaries) through which blood moves, and the heart (a muscular pump, which continually pushes blood through the body).

Around 2 ounces (59 ml) of blood is pumped out of the heart each time it contracts. Blood that is rich in oxygen and nutrients starts its journey from the left side of the heart, through a large artery called the aorta. The blood flows from the aorta through arteries into smaller vessels called arterioles, which supply the body's tissues. From the arterioles, blood enters a network of minute vessels called capillaries. Oxygen and nutrients are transferred to cells, and carbon dioxide and waste products are absorbed.

Deoxygenated blood then flows from the capillaries into small veins (venules) to return to the heart. The veins eventually merge into two large blood vessels, the venae cavae. From here, deoxygenated blood is delivered to the right side of the heart, pumped into the pulmonary artery, and taken to the lungs. Fresh oxygen is absorbed into the blood and the waste carbon dioxide is expelled from the body by breathing out. The now oxygen-rich blood flows through the pulmonary vein into the left side of the heart, and the journey through the body begins all over again. This complete circuit takes about 60 seconds. The heart beats on average 70 times every minute. It pumps an estimated 8,000 gallons (30,280 l) of blood around the body every 24 hours.

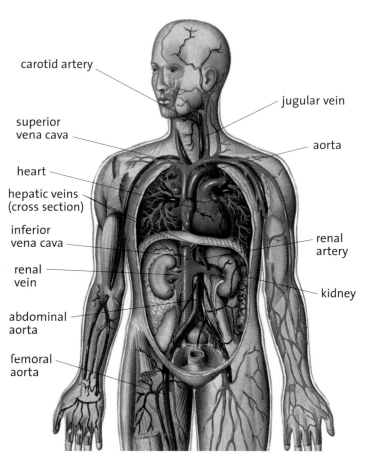

carotid artery

jugular vein

superior vena cava

aorta

heart

hepatic veins (cross section)

inferior vena cava

renal artery

renal vein

kidney

abdominal aorta

femoral aorta

The circulatory system's main arteries (red) and veins (blue) would cover many thousands of miles if they were removed from the body and laid out.

SEE ALSO

BLOOD PRESSURE • BODY SYSTEMS • HEART • OXYGEN • RESPIRATORY SYSTEM

Coffee and Tea

Most people drink coffee or tea. A cup of either drink may wake them up in the morning or perk them up when they feel tired. Too much coffee and tea, however, is not always a good thing. Both beverages contain the mild stimulant caffeine. Caffeine acts on the central nervous system. It stimulates the brain and muscles and acts on the heart, blood vessels, and kidneys. In large amounts, it can cause insomnia (sleeplessness), restlessness, nervousness, a rapid pulse, and ringing in the ears. Caffeine also encourages the production of acid in the stomach and can cause indigestion and gastric acidity. In addition to caffeine, tea contains tannin (which can cause constipation) and theophylline (a stimulant that increases heart rate and acts on the kidneys as a diuretic, a substance that increases the output of urine by the kidneys).

Small doses

Tea and coffee have limited food value, although they do contain vitamin B and folic acid, which help prevent anemia. In small amounts, tea and coffee are unlikely to do harm. However, people suffering from indigestion, stomach ulcers, or nervousness should limit the amount they drink. In addition, people with diabetes, coronary disease, or hypertension should avoid tea and coffee.

Q & A

Is coffee really a kind of stimulant?

Yes. Coffee has a nonspecific stimulating action on the brain. This effect is produced by the action of caffeine, which is present in both coffee and tea. Many people find coffee so effective at stimulating the arousal system that they cannot drink it in the evening, because it prevents sleep.

CAFFEINE

Coffee and tea are not the only substances that contain caffeine. Cocoa and cola drinks that are made from the kola nut also contain caffeine and related compounds. If people want to avoid caffeine, they can drink decaffeinated coffee, herbal teas, and a whole range of caffeine-free drinks that are now available.

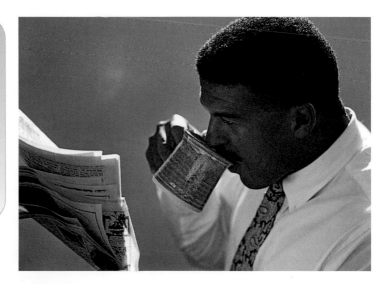

Many people find that a cup of coffee helps wake them up so that they feel ready to start the day.

SEE ALSO

ANEMIA • AUTONOMIC NERVOUS SYSTEM • BLOOD PRESSURE • DIABETES • NERVOUS SYSTEM

Constipation

Most people open their bowels at regular intervals, usually once or twice a day or perhaps once every two days. If a person's normal pattern changes and an unusually long time between bowel movements is experienced, and the stools are difficult or painful to pass, then the person is suffering from constipation. As a result, the abdomen becomes swollen and the sufferer may also have a furred tongue with white discoloration, gas, bad breath, and even headaches.

Normally, food is moved along the intestines by regular muscle action called peristalsis. Constipation occurs when something interferes with these actions: for example, eating the wrong foods or not enough food. Some people find they become constipated if their normal routine is altered: for example, when they go on vacation. Lack of exercise and taking certain drugs can also cause constipation. Serious diseases such as colitis and diverticulitis can also result in constipation.

Constipation accompanied by pain on defecation tends to create a spiral of problems. The pain, which is commonly due to hemorrhoids (damaged veins) or cracks (fissures) in the anus, causes a reluctance to defecate. That makes the feces collect in the rectum, where more water is absorbed from them, and they become harder and even more painful to pass.

Q & A

Why do I always get constipated when I am on vacation?

Many people blame "vacation constipation" on a change in the water, but it is more likely to be due to the change in your routine or to the stress of traveling. Even using a strange toilet can be a problem, especially if it is a different height from the one you are used to or has an unusual smell that makes you reluctant to obey your body's command to defecate.

My father finally gave up smoking, but now I hear him complaining about being constipated. Why would giving up smoking cause constipation?

The nicotine in tobacco smoke tends to speed up the movement of food through the digestive system and stimulate defecation. It is the withdrawal of the drug that has made your father constipated. He should ensure he gets a high-roughage diet, plenty of fluids, and regular exercise.

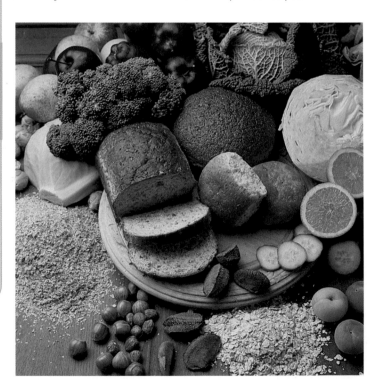

Fresh fruits, vegetables, and bran help relieve constipation. They should be included in everyone's regular diet.

CAUSES OF CONSTIPATION

Cause	Additional symptoms	Treatment
Persistent ignoring of signals telling the brain that the bowel is full	Headache, furred tongue, gas, bad breath, distended and possibly painful abdomen	Try to set aside a regular time for using the toilet each day; increase the fiber content of the regular diet.
Persistent use of chemical laxatives that can inhibit the colon's natural function	As above	Stop taking laxatives unless prescribed by a doctor; eat a high-fiber diet; drink more fluids; exercise more.
Muscle weakness in old age or after having a baby	As above	Change to a diet as above, but if the problem persists, see a doctor.
Reducing food intake, anorexia nervosa, low food intake due to mental or physical illness	As above, plus symptoms of underlying cause of illness	If it is due to a reducing diet, take two tablespoons of bran daily (contains no calories). Otherwise, see a doctor for treatment of the underlying cause.
Obsession with bowel movements, anxiety or stress about constipation.	May be accompanied by furred tongue, gas, and other symptoms of constipation	Try to ignore bowel movements and change to a high-fiber diet; drink more fluids and get more exercise.
Damage to anus; hemorrhoids (piles)	Painful defecation, hard bowel movements, possibly bleeding from anus, causing tendency to "hold back"	Consult a doctor, as drugs and possibly surgery may be needed to treat the problem, rather than self-help.
Intestinal obstruction due to twisting or constriction of intestine	Vomiting, acute pain in abdomen	Medical emergency; get to the hospital as quickly as possible.
Diverticulitis (formation and inflammation of small extensions from the colon)	Pain in lower left abdomen, temperature may be raised	See a doctor as soon as possible; make a long-term change to a high-fiber diet.

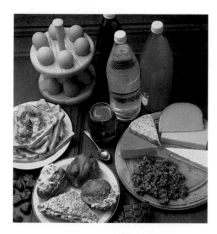

A badly balanced diet with too many creamy and sugary foods such as these can cause constipation.

Treatment

Except when constipation is caused by a psychological or mental illness, the best treatment is common sense. Eating a fiber-rich diet helps avoid or cure constipation. Fresh fruits and vegetables and cereals containing bran are excellent fiber sources. Exercising also helps, because it tones the abdominal muscles and provides relaxation from stress. Laxatives should not be taken unless prescribed by a doctor. These drugs work by irritating the nerves of the intestines and speeding up peristalsis. They may cause pains and the passing of semiliquid feces.

SEE ALSO

DIET • DIETING • DIGESTIVE SYSTEM • DIGESTIVE SYSTEM DISEASES AND DISORDERS

Cramps

A cramp is a sudden and often severe pain, caused by the contraction of a muscle or group of muscles. Cramps are common in the legs—in the muscles of the calf or in the back of the thigh. The muscles contract into a hard knot, and ordinary efforts to move the muscles and relax them are useless. The cramp comes on suddenly, sometimes when the person is asleep, and may last from a few seconds to several minutes.

There are various causes of cramps: for example, poor circulation, which prevents enough blood from getting to the muscles; and sitting or lying in an uncomfortable position. Cold and exhaustion can also cause cramps. Heat can lead to sweating and the loss of salt from the body. That, in turn, leads to cramps. Another cause of cramps is unusual or hard exercise, particularly if a person has eaten immediately before exercising. It is particularly important not to eat for at least half an hour before swimming; cramps have caused many swimmers to drown. Some people who work with their hands, such as writers, artists, and musicians, suffer from hand cramps, and women may have menstrual cramps at the start of a period.

An attack of cramps can be helped by first stretching and then massaging the muscles. Bending the foot upward may help ease the pain of a leg cramp. Food containing salt will both prevent and relieve salt-deficiency cramps. Salt tablets are available but they can cause stomach irritation. People who suffer from persistent cramps should check with a doctor to be sure that they are not a symptom of a circulatory problem.

Q & A

My brother says he suffers from writer's cramp. What is it?

Writer's cramp is also known as professional or occupational cramp. It can affect people who use their hands for delicate work, such as musicians, seamstresses, and artists, as well as writers. The muscles of the fingers, and even the forearm, seize, so that work with the affected hand is impossible.

My mother is pregnant and frequently suffers from cramps in her legs at night. Why is this?

Your mother's muscles are under additional strain during the day, owing to the unaccustomed weight of the developing baby. As a result, they go into spasm at night when she is lying down and relaxed. You can help her by massaging her legs when the cramp occurs, because she will not be able to reach them comfortably herself. Once she has had the baby, it is likely that the attacks will disappear.

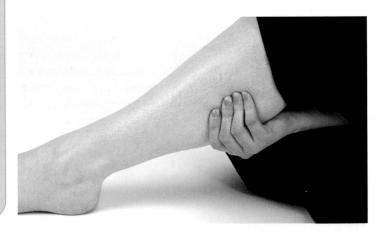

A cramp in the calf muscle can usually be relieved by massaging the muscle, flexing the foot upward, and walking around for a while.

SEE ALSO

CIRCULATORY SYSTEM • EXERCISE • MUSCLE • PAIN • SALT

54

Diabetes

Diabetes mellitus is a disease in which the body does not produce sufficient amounts of the hormone insulin. This hormone directs the body's sugar into the cells, where it is used as fuel. Without insulin, the cells cannot work properly. Insulin-dependent diabetes, or type 1 diabetes, is quite a common illness. It used to be fatal, but modern treatments allow diabetics (people with diabetes) to lead normal lives.

Symptoms of diabetes

Diabetes can start at any age. It often begins abruptly in children but progresses more gradually in adults. The body either stops producing insulin or makes so little that it is unable to work properly. The most obvious symptom is a great thirst, causing people with diabetes to drink a large amount and produce a lot of urine. They also feel tired and weak because their body is not getting enough fuel. They may have blurred vision and itching skin, and because their resistance is low, they are vulnerable to all kinds of infections.

People with diabetes lose weight quickly, as their body uses up their fat as a fuel to replace sugar. This in turn produces harmful waste products that can cause a diabetic to go into a coma and to die. A doctor can easily tell when someone has diabetes, because the blood and urine both contain unusually large amounts of sugar.

Treatment of diabetes

People with severe diabetes treat themselves with daily injections of insulin. Diabetics are shown how to administer this themselves. Even young children are able to inject themselves. Doctors figure out how much insulin each person needs to function properly. The dose must be balanced with the person's intake of sugar and carbohydrates, so a diabetic must eat carefully and at regular times.

Getting the balance right is extremely important; if the blood sugar falls too low, the diabetic can go into insulin shock, known as hypoglycemia. The patient feels hungry, then dizzy, and soon loses consciousness. Someone who feels an attack coming on should eat something sweet as quickly as possible to raise the blood sugar. Diabetics should carry sugar lumps, candy, or other sweet foods with them at all times to counter such an attack.

People with mild diabetes may be able to control the condition by eating carefully and keeping their weight within a reasonable range. They must be particularly careful not to eat too much sugar or food containing sugar. They may also need tablets to make their bodies produce more insulin.

Q & A

I think my little brother eats far too much candy. All that sugar can't be good for him. Won't it cause him to develop diabetes—either now or later in life?

No. If a child is going to get diabetes, it will be the type caused by the failure to produce insulin (a hormone produced in the pancreas). Being overweight or eating sweet things has nothing to do with whether the insulin-producing cells in the pancreas are functioning properly or not.

My father has recently been diagnosed as having diabetes. I am afraid the illness may change his personality, by making him bad-tempered, for example. Am I right to worry about this?

Not really. Obviously, diabetes, like any illness, can put the patient under strain, but it does not cause personality changes. There is certainly nothing to suggest that diabetic children develop inadequate personalities because of their diabetes as they grow up.

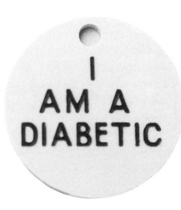

It is a good idea for people with diabetes to wear a tag such as this. If they were to slip into a diabetic coma, the emergency medical service would know immediately that they were diabetic, and precious time would be saved.

Checking urine and blood

Diabetics check their urine or blood regularly to make sure that the sugar level is correct. The only really effective way to control blood sugar is to check the levels in the blood at regular intervals. That is done using a small monitoring device that can determine blood sugar levels in blood taken from a small prick in the finger. Careful diabetic control reduces the risk of later complications.

Noninsulin-dependent diabetes

Not all diabetics need insulin injections, but for those not taking insulin it is essential to ensure that the body's own insulin production is adequate. Noninsulin-dependent diabetes (NIDD)—also known as type 2 diabetes or maturity-onset diabetes—can have serious complications. Insulin is still produced by the pancreas, but in quantities insufficient for the body's overall needs.

Noninsulin-dependent diabetes usually starts between the ages of 50 and 65, although it can affect people as young as 15. It may occur in people older than 65, and it may also have a genetic factor and run in families; of every three people with NIDD, approximately one has a relative who is also affected with the disorder. This type of diabetes usually starts with insulin resistance, a condition in which the cells cannot use insulin properly. At first, more insulin is made to compensate, but eventually the pancreas loses the ability to secrete insulin.

A principal, but not the sole, cause of NIDD is obesity. About 80 percent of people with NIDD are obese. For reasons that are not fully understood, obesity is associated with a state known as insulin resistance. It may simply be that the number of insulin receptor sites is inadequate, or it may be that the mechanisms triggered in the cell by insulin locking are adversely affected. It is known that people in wealthier societies tend to eat more food, which leads to a rise in obesity and hence a rise in NIDD.

Controlling NIDD

The object of treatment is to keep blood sugar levels within normal limits so that complications do not occur. Exercise and a healthy diet to maintain an appropriate weight are important in controlling blood sugar levels. In many cases, NIDD can be completely controlled by diet alone. What is eaten is just as important as how much is eaten. The aim is to control the blood sugar without drugs, but if necessary, production of insulin can be boosted by sulfonylurea drugs such as tolbutamide, chlorpropamide, or other drugs. If these drugs fail, insulin injections will then become necessary.

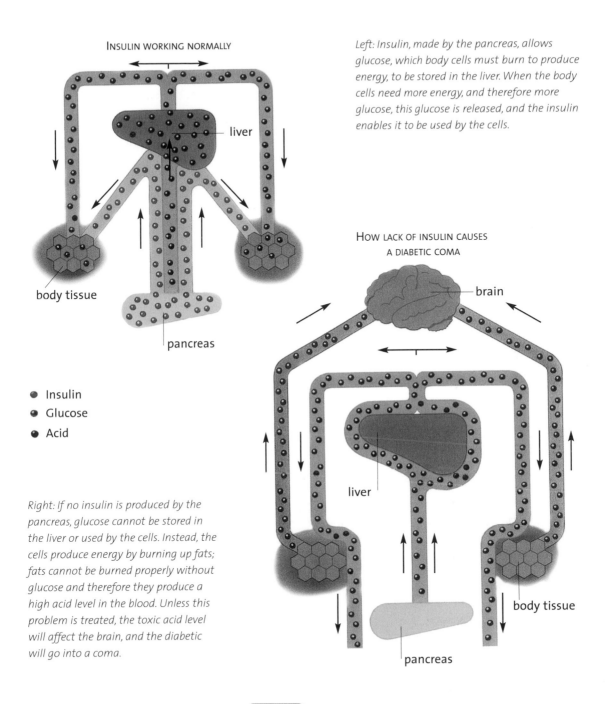

INSULIN WORKING NORMALLY

liver

body tissue

pancreas

- Insulin
- Glucose
- Acid

Left: Insulin, made by the pancreas, allows glucose, which body cells must burn to produce energy, to be stored in the liver. When the body cells need more energy, and therefore more glucose, this glucose is released, and the insulin enables it to be used by the cells.

HOW LACK OF INSULIN CAUSES
A DIABETIC COMA

brain

liver

body tissue

pancreas

Right: If no insulin is produced by the pancreas, glucose cannot be stored in the liver or used by the cells. Instead, the cells produce energy by burning up fats; fats cannot be burned properly without glucose and therefore they produce a high acid level in the blood. Unless this problem is treated, the toxic acid level will affect the brain, and the diabetic will go into a coma.

SEE ALSO

CARBOHYDRATES • CIRCULATORY SYSTEM • DIET • OBESITY •
SUGARS • TIREDNESS

Diet

The body is like an engine, and food is the fuel it needs to keep running. How efficiently the body works depends on what is consumed. The food a person eats is changed into energy and used by the body for different functions, such as walking and running and the constant process of growth and repair of the body tissues. The amount of energy (and therefore the amount of food) needed depends on how much energy is used; on the type of activities performed; and on body size, sex, age, and general health. Figures given for the needs of a person at rest are known as the basal metabolic rate. Every person must eat the right amount of food to fuel his or her needs. If more food is eaten than is needed, the excess is stored as fat and the person becomes overweight.

Carbohydrates, proteins, and fats

Food can be divided into three main types: carbohydrates, proteins, and fats. Carbohydrates are present in starch (potatoes, bread, yams, peas, corn, beans) and sugar (fruit, honey, table sugar). Sugar-rich foods include jams, cookies, chocolate, candy, and ice cream. Meat, fish, eggs, cheese, milk, soybeans, nuts, some pulses, lentils, and seeds are rich sources of protein. Carbohydrates and fats are used to fuel the body's processes and functions; protein is used as building material for the tissues, including muscles and bones. Fats provide nearly three times as much energy as other foods, so fewer of them are needed in the diet. In the West, people eat far too much fat. About 40 percent of their energy comes from fats, and this situation has led to high levels of obesity and diseases of the arteries and the heart.

Vitamins, minerals, and roughage

The body needs vitamins A, B, C, D, E, and K and minerals such as calcium, phosphorus, iron, iodine, potassium, magnesium, fluorine, zinc, and copper. Vitamins are essential for normal growth and development, and because they cannot be made by the body, they must be included in the diet. Vitamins can be taken as supplements. Minerals assist in many of the processes needed for normal nerve and muscle function and must be supplied frequently in the diet.

Roughage, or dietary fiber, consists of the walls of plant cells that cannot be broken down by digestion and therefore pass through the stomach and intestine in solid form. Roughage stimulates the action of the intestine and enables food to pass through the digestive system more easily. It also provides the bulk to make feces solid. The best-known example of roughage is bran. Vegetables, nuts, and cereals also contain fiber.

The five food groups in the MyPyramid diet are grains (orange band), half of which should be whole grains; vegetables (green band); fruits (red band), which can be fresh, canned, frozen, or dried; milk products (blue band), preferably low-fat or fat-free; and meat and beans (purple band), mainly lean meat and poultry, fish, beans, nuts, and seeds. The wider the band, the more that food should be eaten daily. The narrow yellow band represents oils (fats), which should be eaten sparingly. Experts recommend that a diet should be low in fats, cholesterol, salt, and added sugars. One of the aims of this pyramid is to highlight the vital health benefits of making small, simple improvements in nutrition, physical activity, and lifestyle behavior.

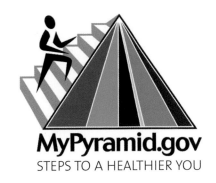

MyPyramid.gov
STEPS TO A HEALTHIER YOU

■	grains	■	vegetables	■	fruits
■	oils	■	milk products	■	meat and beans

A balanced diet and food pyramids

A balanced diet supplies all the necessary nutrients in quantities that suit a particular individual. The original food guide pyramid recommended that people should eat plenty of whole-grain foods, vegetables, and fruits and fewer high-fat, high-sugar foods. In 2005, the United States Department of Agriculture (USDA) updated the old food pyramid and put forward new guidance in the form of "MyPyramid: Steps to a Healthier You." This system was designed to help people make healthier food choices and to be active every day.

The old food pyramid has been turned on its side so that all the food group bands now run from the top of the pyramid to the base. The different size of each band shows the proportion from each food group that should be eaten each day. The wider the band at the base, the more of that food should be eaten every day. The emphasis is on a high-fiber, low-fat diet.

The steps at the side of the new pyramid are to encourage people to be active every day. There are 12 different pyramids to choose from, depending on how many calories a person needs and how active he or she is. This emphasizes the need for a more personal and individualized approach to improving diet and lifestyle. One pyramid is aimed at children to help show them the importance of healthy eating and physical activity and to address the very serious problem of childhood obesity.

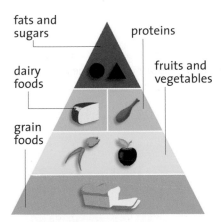

fats and sugars

proteins

dairy foods

fruits and vegetables

grain foods

The original food guide pyramid emphasized the importance of eating more foods in the blue and yellow bands and fewer in the green and red bands.

SEE ALSO

BASAL METABOLISM • CARBOHYDRATES • DIETING • FATS • FOOD AND NUTRITION • HEALTH FOODS • OBESITY • PROTEIN • SUGARS • VITAMINS • WEIGHT CONTROL

Dieting

The most common reason for dieting is being overweight. People put on excess weight because they are taking in more energy (calories) in their food than they are using. Obesity—being more than 30 percent above the ideal body weight—is reaching epidemic proportions in the United States and in other developed countries. Obesity is a serious risk to health; it can lead to heart disease, high blood pressure, and diabetes.

There are no hard-and-fast rules about how much people should eat and drink. Some people can consume what they like and still stay slim; other people gain weight on an apparently normal diet. The difference happens because the rate at which a person's body uses energy—the metabolic rate—varies from one individual to another.

Healthy choices and exercise

People who want to lose weight need to cut down on the amount they eat, but they should still eat a balanced diet that includes lean meat, poultry, fish, fresh fruits and vegetables, whole-grain bread, brown rice, and low-fat milk products, such as spreads and cheeses. They should also avoid or cut down drastically on food containing a high proportion of sugar and fat, such as cookies, candy, cake, french fries, hamburgers, salami, and fried food. Neither should they eat too much protein

Q & A

I want to lose weight, but I'm confused by all the different diets and their claims. I am looking for a simple and effective way to lose weight. What should I do?

A reducing diet allows for around 1,000 calories a day. It should include a variety of foods low in fat and plenty of cooked or raw vegetables, fresh fruits, meats, and grain products. Try to avoid using salt and excess sugar.

I've decided that I need to go on a diet. Can I still eat as much as I want of foods that are advertised as being "low-fat"? If not, why?

No. Even if a product is advertised as having zero fat, it can still contain lots of calories. In fact, in a product that is fat-free, manufacturers have often replaced the fat with sugar. Always check the food's calorie content on the nutrition label.

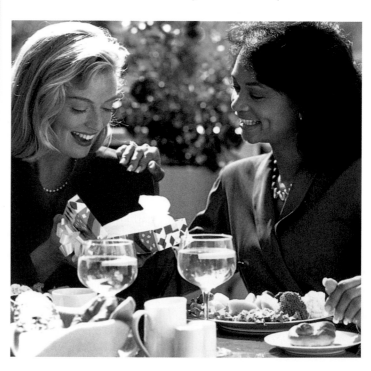

Eating plenty of fresh fruits and vegetables and drinking water rather than sweet drinks or alcohol keeps these two women slim and healthy.

CUT DOWN ON

- Butter, cream, and ice cream
- High-calorie cheese
- Fatty meats such as bacon, hamburgers, and salami
- Fried foods
- Desserts, cakes, cookies, and pies
- Chocolate and candy
- Dried nuts
- Thick sauces
- Sweet drinks

INSTEAD EAT

- Whole wheat bread
- Brown rice
- Pasta
- Vegetables
- Fruit
- Skim milk
- Lean beef, lamb, and pork
- Chicken and turkey
- Dry beans
- Whitefish

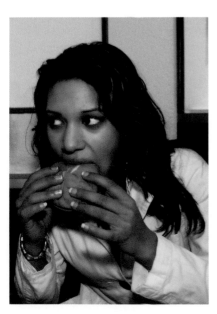

containing saturated fat, because that increases the body's production of unhealthy cholesterol. Dry beans, peas, and lentils are good sources of low-fat vegetable protein, and when combined with grains, these pulses make a good meat substitute. The MyPyramid food guidance system put forward in 2005 by the United States Department of Agriculture (USDA) is designed to help people make healthier food choices and emphasizes the importance of physical activity in keeping one's weight at a healthy level.

People who are dieting should not cut out meals completely. If they try to get through the day without eating, they will find themselves filling up later with junk food. They should eat three small meals a day and cut out sugary snacks. If they must eat between meals, they should nibble a celery stick or an apple.

Eating too much salt is bad because it makes the body retain more fluid. Cutting down on salt allows the body to eliminate fluid, and this loss of fluid makes a person slimmer. It is best not to cut down on the amount of liquid consumed; drinking less has no effect on weight. The only liquids that should be cut out are sweet drinks and alcohol; drinks containing caffeine should be limited.

Permanent changes

One of the keys to successful dieting is a genuine desire to lose weight. The type of diet that is followed is also an important factor. All kinds of diets come into and out of fashion. Some diets suggest that only one type of food, for example bananas, should be eaten for several days; others rely on special packaged diet meals that claim to contain all the nourishment needed. Neither type of diet, however, is likely to provide sufficient nutrients. Many people go on crash diets and lose several pounds quickly. Dieting, however, is not just a matter of losing weight. It also involves not putting weight on again. Many dieters lose weight on a crash diet and then go back to their old eating habits. Before long, they put all the weight back on.

The best way to lose weight is not to diet at all but to change eating habits permanently. By eating sensibly and altering the proportions of the foods that are eaten each day, a person should be able to lose 1 pound (450 g) a week. In six months, that will equal a weight loss of about 25 pounds (11 kg). This weight loss can be achieved on a diet that is interesting, is balanced, and

Foods such as hamburgers and fries are popular, but they should be avoided or eaten sparingly, because they contain extremely high levels of fats and sugar. Consequently, their calorie content is very high.

A fruit smoothie, such as this banana smoothie, is a healthy snack that is low in calories, sugar, and fat. It contains only nonfat yogurt, a banana, crushed ice, and a little honey.

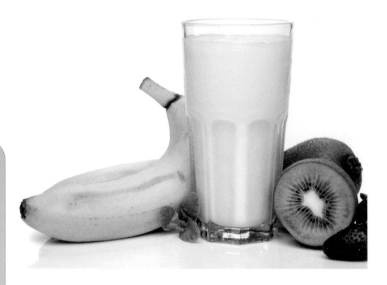

SPECIAL DIETS

Doctors prescribe special diets as part of the treatment for some diseases, such as liver and kidney disorders, hypertension (high blood pressure), gastrointestinal disturbances, and diabetes.

Kidney and liver illnesses may be treated with a protein-free diet, consisting largely of bland, sweet puddings and unsalted butter. This is a short-term diet, however, to be used in emergencies only.

Patients with hypertension are often put on a low-salt, low-cholesterol diet, which reduces or cuts out all animal fats, dairy products, eggs, and candy.

Gastrointestinal disturbances are made worse by any diet containing too much fiber, so people with severe cases should avoid high-fiber foods, such as whole-wheat breads and cereals, nuts and legumes (peas, beans), and most raw fruits and vegetables.

Diabetics must keep strictly to a diet that contains fixed amounts of calories and carbohydrates; unless they adhere to this, they may lose consciousness and go into a coma.

does not leave the person feeling hungry. Such a dieting method does not mean eating different food from other people. It means avoiding certain foods; eating less of some, more of others; and generally eating slightly less.

Weight-loss groups and counseling

Many people find it helpful to join a weight-loss group in which dieters encourage one another and exchange helpful tips. They can discuss their problems, work out a sensible diet that suits each invidual, and have fun exercising with friends. If someone finds losing weight difficult, he or she should consult a counselor who will be able to advise and help. If someone falls short of a weight-loss target, he or she should not be discouraged but keep trying. When people have lost as much weight as they want, they can keep their weight at the new level by continuing to eat a balanced diet, joining in sports activitles, and exercising regularly.

As people lose weight, they should check themselves regularly once a week against weight-for-height charts. They should ensure that they do not fall below the ideal weight range. Being too thin is as undesirable as being too fat and is also unhealthy. People who are worried about being too heavy or too thin should talk to a counselor, teacher, or doctor.

SEE ALSO

ANOREXIA AND BULIMIA • BASAL METABOLISM • DIABETES • DIET • EXERCISE • FOOD AND NUTRITION • FOOD LABELING • OBESITY • WEIGHT CONTROL

Digestive System

The digestive system is the part of the body that breaks down food into a form that can be absorbed by the cells. The digestive tract is sometimes called the alimentary canal. It consists of the mouth, throat, esophagus, stomach, and intestines.

From mouth to stomach

In the digestive system, digestive juices called enzymes act on the food that is eaten. Organs connected with the digestive tract produce these enzymes. Digestion begins in the mouth. As food is chewed, glands beneath the tongue increase the production of saliva, which contains the enzyme ptyalin. This enzyme starts breaking down some of the carbohydrates in the food into glucose and maltose, which are simple sugars.

From the mouth, the food travels through the throat and down the esophagus, or gullet. There, the gastric juices—a mixture of secretions composed of mucus, hydrochloric acid, and another enzyme, pepsin—are mixed with the food. The gastric juices in the stomach start to work on the proteins (foods such as eggs, cheese, chicken, and meat). The muscles in the walls of the stomach knead and churn the food around to aid digestion.

The small intestine, pancreas, and gallbladder

About four and a half hours after swallowing food, the partially digested mixture leaves the stomach in the form of a thickish, acidic liquid called chyme. This liquid passes into the duodenum, the first part of the small intestine, which is a coiled tube about 20 feet (6 m) long. The duodenum is the first part of the small intestine, which is about 10 inches (25 cm) long. Chyme contains a quantity of acid and enzymes that could damage the duodenum, but the duodenum plays a vital part in digestion by making and releasing large quantities of mucus, which protect the lining. The alkaline duodenal juices are produced under the influence of the hormone secretin, which helps neutralize the acids in the chyme.

The pancreas and the gallbladder also help with digestion. In response to the presence of food in the upper digestive tract, the gallbladder adds more enzymes that break down fats, nucleic acids, proteins, and carbohydrates. Bile is released via the bile ducts from the gallbladder, where it is stored. Bile is a yellowish fluid secreted by the liver, which helps digest fats.

From the duodenum, the partially digested food passes into the rest of the small intestine. The food takes nearly three hours to pass through the long, narrow tube of the small intestine. During its passage, the food is broken down completely by a series of enzymes. Amylase converts starch into maltose; lipase converts fats into glycerin and fatty acids; and trypsin reduces

Q & A

Is it true that babies can't digest cow's milk?

Compared with human breast milk, cow's milk contains large amounts of a protein called casein, which babies do not have the equipment to digest properly. The many powdered formula milks for babies are made from cow's milk and thus contain more casein than breast milk, but the formula milks are specially treated to make the casein more digestible. However, breast-feeding is better for a baby's digestive system, and in other ways, too.

My three-year-old sister loves spicy foods. However, won't they upset her stomach and her digestion?

There is no reason why spicy foods should cause her any problems. By the age of three, a child's digestive system can cope with an extremely mixed diet, and the degree of tolerance to spicy foods will vary, just as it does in adults. As long as these foods do not give her diarrhea or make her vomit, let her have foods that she likes.

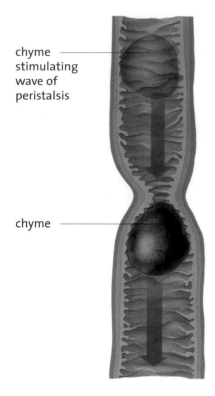

chyme stimulating wave of peristalsis

chyme

Partially digested food (chyme) is moved through the intestine in waves, as the walls of the intestine contract and then relax. This wave movement is called peristalsis. It is stimulated by the presence of food in the esophagus.

proteins to amino acids. More enzymes are released from the walls of the small intestine to complete digestion. The broken-down food is now ready to be absorbed into the bloodstream.

Absorbing nutrients

The lining of the small intestine contains millions of minute projections called villi. Each villus is covered by a cell layer that absorbs nutrients. These cells have projections called microvilli. Both the villi and the microvilli increase the surface area of the small intestine to enable the efficient absorption of nutrients. The central core of each villus contains a capillary (a small blood vessel) and lacteals, which are branches of the lymphatic system. This system is a network of tiny tubes (the lymph vessels) carrying lymph, which is normally a colorless fluid. After a fatty meal, the lymph in the lacteals is milky white, owing to the presence of tiny fat globules. The function of the lymphatic system is to return liquid to the bloodstream. When digested food comes into contact with the villi, the glycerols, fatty acids, and dissolved vitamins enter the lacteals and travel through the lymphatic system to enter the bloodstream.

Other substances are absorbed directly into the capillaries in the villi. These substances include amino acids from protein digestion; sugars from carbohydrates; vitamins; and important minerals such as calcium, iodine, and iron. From the capillaries, these substances go to the liver, which extracts some of them. The rest go into the general blood circulation and are taken to the cells to provide them with energy.

The large intestine

When the digested food has gone through the small intestine, the remainder passes into the large intestine, or colon, as waste. The colon extracts water from the waste, which collects in the rectum and passes out through the anus as feces.

The surface of the small intestine is covered with small, fingerlike projections called villi. They increase the surface area and allow food to be absorbed quickly into the capillaries (blood vessels).

villi

capillaries

lymph vessels

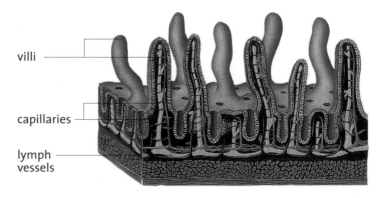

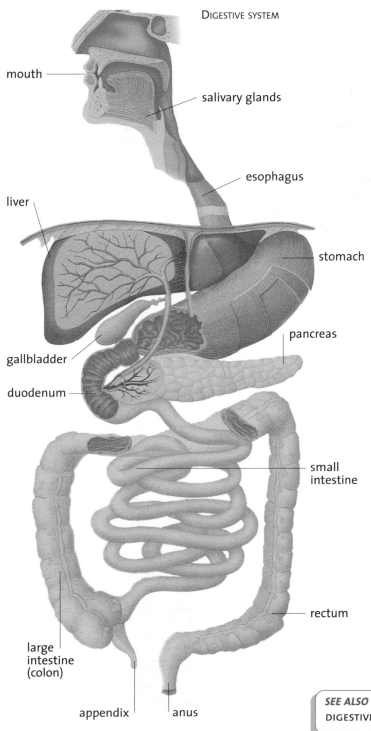

DIGESTIVE SYSTEM

mouth

salivary glands

esophagus

liver

stomach

pancreas

gallbladder

duodenum

small intestine

large intestine (colon)

rectum

appendix

anus

MOUTH *Food is taken into the mouth.*

SALIVARY GLANDS *They produce saliva, which moistens the food while the enzymes it contains start digestion.*

ESOPHAGUS *Waves of muscle action called peristalsis move the food down the esophagus, or gullet, and into the stomach.*

STOMACH *In the stomach, the food is mixed with digestive juices. After two to six hours, it is converted to a liquid called chyme.*

SMALL INTESTINE *Waves of peristalsis push chyme through the stomach and out in small amounts into the small intestine. The small intestine of an adult measures approximately 20 feet (6 m) long and 1.5 inches (4 cm) wide. Most of the digestive process happens here.*

LIVER AND PANCREAS *The liver and pancreas produce digestive juices.*

LARGE INTESTINE *Chyme passes from the small intestine into the large intestine, which is about 3 inches (7.5 cm) in diameter and 3 feet (1 m) long. The appendix leads off the large intestine.*

COLON *The greater part of the large intestine is known as the colon. As chyme passes through the colon, water is absorbed into the blood.*

RECTUM *In the rectum, only solid feces remain. They are pushed out through the anus by deliberate muscle contractions.*

SEE ALSO
DIGESTIVE SYSTEM DISEASES AND DISORDERS

Digestive System Diseases and Disorders

Q & A

My mother says that laxatives are dangerous and that you should always treat constipation naturally. Is she right, and what does she mean by "naturally"?

Yes, your mother is right. Too many laxatives can harm your digestive system. The best natural remedies for constipation are bran, fresh fruits, and vegetables. These foods contain the naturally occurring substances, especially fiber, that encourage the bowels to move regularly, without harming them.

My grandmother got very sick when she was at our house and she had symptoms of diarrhea. However, when the doctor came, he said it was really constipation. How could this be?

This is a rather common ailment in the elderly, called spurious diarrhea. The lower intestine gets clogged with feces, yet some liquid matter manages to get past the blockage, appearing as diarrhea, and may cause the older person to lose control of the bowels and become incontinent. However, this problem can be easily treated.

Many digestive disorders are caused by the food people eat. The digestive system works best when people eat a diet containing a good deal of fiber and not too much fat. A low-fiber diet can cause constipation (infrequent bowel movements, with small, hard stools), and eating extremely spicy food can cause diarrhea, if people are not accustomed to such food.

Indigestion, or dyspepsia, can be caused by nervousness, eating too fast, and emotional stress. It results in discomfort, belching, and heartburn. Also associated with indigestion is flatulence, which is a buildup of gas in the intestines. Sensible eating habits and relaxation are the most common treatments for indigestion.

Contaminated food and appendicitis

Some painful and dangerous illnesses are caused by eating food contaminated by bacteria, including staphylococcal poisoning, salmonella poisoning, amebic and bacillary dysentery, botulism, cholera, and typhoid fever. These illnesses cause many symptoms, inlcuding vomiting, abdominal pain, and diarrhea. Foods may be contaminated by chemicals, which cause vomiting, or be poisonous themselves, as are some fungi.

Appendicitis is inflammation of the appendix, normally as a result of bacterial infection. It is most common between the ages of 15 and 24 years. The symptoms include pain in the lower right abdomen and sometimes nausea and vomiting. Treatment involves surgery to remove the appendix.

Ulcers and inflammation

Ulcers are small, open sores that form when the mucous membrane lining the digestive tract is damaged. Small ulcers often form in the mouth but heal quickly. Ulcers in the stomach and duodenum are more serious. Although the exact cause is unclear, the bacterium *Helicobacter pylori* may cause inflammation and ulceration by increasing stomach acid. Ulcers are more common in people who eat hurried and irregular meals, who drink heavily, who smoke, or who are nervous and under stress.

Inflammation, thickening, and ulceration of the colon or another region of the digestive tract can cause Crohn's disease, with cramps and pains after eating. There may be persistent diarrhea, abdominal pain, fever, loss of weight, and bleeding, leading to anemia. Drugs can relieve the anemia, but surgery may be needed. Inflammations and ulcerations of the colon are called colitis. Some inflammations are caused by an infection or an allergy and last a short time, but others are chronic

GASTROINTESTINAL DISORDERS

Disorder	Symptoms	Treatment
Bad breath (halitosis): Unpleasant odor due to swallowed food or drink, dental disease, or sometimes disorders of the respiratory or digestive systems	Bad breath	Removal of cause, change of diet, and good dental hygiene
Foreign bodies: Fish bones, toothpicks, buttons, coins, and so on, swallowed by children and the unwary	Choking, or severe pain in colon	Small round objects can pass through the digestive tract with no problem. Sharper ones may require surgery.
Gastritis: Inflammation of the stomach lining, caused by drugs, food poisoning, infection, alcohol, or eating the wrong type of food (acute); inflammation of the lining of the stomach, leading to ulceration and hemorrhage, caused by poor diet, alcoholism, enzyme deficiency, hiatus hernia, diabetes, cancer, or emotional stress (chronic)	Pain in abdomen, loss of appetite, nausea, vomiting, and diarrhea (acute gastritis); pain on eating, pain in back, rapid feeling of fullness, nausea, and blood in vomit (chronic gastritis)	Usually corrects itself when the cause has been eliminated by vomiting or diarrhea; bed rest and bland diet are recommended (acute). Treatment for specific diseases and avoidance of alcohol, tobacco, and very spicy food; bland diet with small meals eaten frequently; removal of causes of stress, or prescription of tranquilizers (chronic)
Gastroenteritis: Inflammation of the lining of the stomach and the intestines	Pain in abdomen, loss of appetite, nausea, vomiting, and diarrhea	As for acute gastritis (above)
Hemorrhoids (piles): Swollen and twisted veins that are located in the anal canal, hemorrhoids may become ulcerated or thrombosed and may eventually protrude from the anus; they occur in most adults.	Pain and bleeding during defecation, constipation	May regress naturally with high-fiber diet; hemorrhoids may be injected, or removed surgically.
Infection and infestation: Bacteria, viruses, and various types of parasites may live in the human digestive tract over a period of time and cause a variety of problems.	Various	Various
Malabsorption: Failure of absorption of nutrients from the digestive tract due to various disorders	Weight loss, increased excretion of protein and fat, diarrhea, and anemia	Various specific diets and treatments
Nausea and vomiting: Vomiting is usually a natural response to harmful substances that must be expelled undigested from the body. Some feelings of nausea and vomiting are psychological in origin.	Nausea due to real or imagined cause; deliberate vomiting during temper tantrums, or on eating wholesome but unpalatable food, or because of an eating disorder	Treatment of physical disorder, if present; reassurance and psychotherapy if not
Peritonitis: Inflammation of the lining of the abdominal cavity and the organs (peritoneum), which is most commonly caused by the perforation or the rupture of an organ such as the appendix, or perforation of an ulcer	Mostly sudden, severe, localized pain in the abdomen, spreading, and leading to shock	Emergency operation, or occasionally medication
Polyps and benign tumors: A growth of protruding tissue that can arise anywhere in the digestive tract	Bleeding, cramps, abdominal pains, or no symptoms	Polyps should be removed by surgery, because some do become cancerous.

conditions. Symptoms are abdominal pain and diarrhea. Chronic colitis may never clear up completely.

One problem of the large intestine is irritable bowel syndrome. Its cause is not really known, but attacks may be triggered by stress. The main symptoms are spasmodic lower abdominal pain and bouts of diarrhea and constipation. A high-fiber diet and antispasmodic drugs may help, but people with irritable bowel syndrome may find it recurs after long gaps, usually when they are nervous or under stress.

Hernias and diverticular disease

The lining of the esophagus is seldom damaged. Sometimes, however, a hiatal hernia forms at the point where the esophagus passes through a gap in the diaphragm and into the abdomen. Part of the esophagus and the upper stomach then bulges back into the chest, and acid from the stomach may make its way back into the esophagus, causing a burning sensation called heartburn. The lining of the esophagus can also be damaged by swallowing acid or a strong alkali.

Sometimes, bulges called diverticula form in the colon, which is the major part of the large intestine. These bulges develop with age, and waste matter may fill them and become infected, causing diverticulitis. The condition can cause bleeding. Alternatively, an inflamed diverticulum may bulge into the abdominal cavity. This extremely serious condition needs immediate surgical treatment. However, rest, a healthy diet, and antibiotics help control diverticulitis.

Cancer of the digestive system

Cancer is unusual in the small intestine but common in the stomach and colon. Treatment may include a combination of surgery, radiotherapy, and chemotherapy. If the disease is diagnosed and treated early enough, patients can live a normal life.

The symptoms are similar for mild or serious cases, so people should consult a doctor if they have long-lasting pain or nausea, if they lose their appetite for more than a few days, if their normal pattern of bowel movements changes, or if they have bleeding.

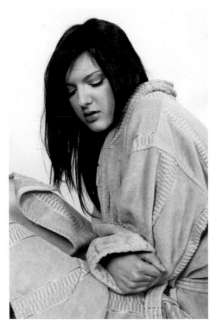

Irritable bowel syndrome results in spasmodic lower abdominal pain and bouts of diarrhea and constipation. Stress and nervousness make it worse.

SEE ALSO

DIGESTIVE SYSTEM • FOOD POISONING • HERNIA • INDIGESTION • IRRITABLE BOWEL SYNDROME • PAIN

Disabilities

A great many people suffer from physical or mental disabilities, or from a combination of both. Sometimes, these disabilities are caused by an inherited condition or by damage at birth. Other disabilities are the result of accidents. A disability may or may not be a handicap; if a disability interferes with a person's capacity to fulfill his or her expectations in life, it is described as a handicap. For example, a ballet dancer is more likely to be handicapped by a limp than a computer operator is.

Born with a disability

Parents of a baby with a disability need help from the very beginning to enable them to come to terms with the problem and to ensure that their baby gets the best possible treatment. There are many voluntary organizations that provide help and advice, and public help may be available as well. There is often a great deal that parents themselves can do to help their child, such as carrying out special exercises and structured play activities. As the child grows up, special schooling may be necessary, either locally, if available, or in a residential center.

Illness and accidents

If people become disabled later in life as the result of an illness or an accident, treatment is based on helping them to do as much as possible for themselves. When possible, disabled people are encouraged to take up sports, which help them improve their physical condition and provide stimulation, self-respect, and fulfillment. It is particularly important that people who are immobile look after their health, as they are often at risk of infection and problems such as pressure sores. People without feeling in a body part are also at risk, because they may hurt themselves badly without realizing it.

Disability aids

All kinds of aids have been developed to make it easier for people with

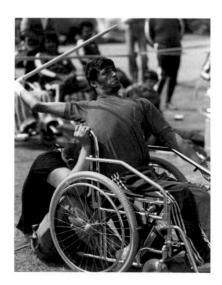

Many people in wheelchairs take up competitive sports, which strengthen their remaining working muscles.

Q & A

My brother has been severely disabled by a car accident and is now confined to a wheelchair. He used to be enthusiastic about sports. How can he continue this interest from a wheelchair?

There are many athletic opportunities for the disabled, such as archery and golf, and many people take part in wheelchair sporting events. You should contact your local association for the disabled, which will be able to give you more information. You can get the address from your public library.

My four-year-old sister is physically challenged and needs my parents a lot. She has to go to the hospital, and I am worried that she won't manage on her own. What can my parents do?

Many hospitals encourage parents to stay in the hospital with their young children. If this is not possible in your sister's case, your parents can visit regularly and explain your sister's likes, dislikes, and needs to the hospital staff.

This diagram shows how an artificial limb works. The wearer can work the elbow joint and hand by moving the stump of his or her arm, the shoulder blades, and the back. The red arrows indicate the movements that can be achieved by using the harness and moving the stump of the limb. The blue arrows indicate the adjustments that are possible by using the other hand.

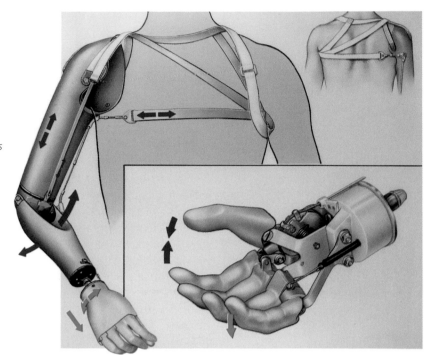

disabilities to lead an independent life. Wheelchairs are constantly being improved and made easier to maneuver, and increasing numbers of stores, hotels, theaters, and offices are designed to give ease of access to wheelchair users. There are also devices such as easy-to-grip faucet handles and computers that enable severely handicapped people to type, answer the telephone, and turn switches on and off, even if the only movement that they are capable of is sucking or blowing through a tube.

Microprocessor technology has been applied to the design of bionic parts, such as arms. These artificial body parts can be activated by tiny electrical signals that originate from the disabled person's own nervous system, so that he or she can perform virtually normal actions.

Elderly people make up the greatest number of the disabled. Most of the effort in treating them medically is devoted to preventing the progress of a disease when possible and alleviating any social and physical distress.

SEE ALSO

MUSCLE • NERVOUS SYSTEM • PARAPLEGIA • STROKE

Drinking Water

The body weight is about two-thirds water. Water is essential to enable the body's delicate chemical processes to take place. An adult loses around 4 pints (1.9 l) of water every day in breath, feces, sweat, and urine. Part of that water is replaced in food (which is 70 percent water); the rest is replaced by drinking. People are unlikely to live for more than a few days if they have nothing at all to eat or drink, but they can survive for about two months without food if they have enough to drink.

The only fluid needed is water; most people take it in the form of drinks such as coffee, milk, soft drinks, or tea. In hot weather, people need to drink more than usual. However, it can be harmful to drink too much water. A healthy body carefully regulates its water content. People experience thirst when the body needs water. Excess water is excreted in the urine.

If the body loses too much water, dehydration occurs. The symptoms include dry skin, weakening muscles, kidney problems, disorientation, and hallucinations. When people have a fever, they perspire more and often eat less. As a result, they may become dehydrated, especially if they vomit and have diarrhea. Those with a fever or upset stomach need to drink lots of fluids.

In some parts of the world, drinking water supplies may carry serious diseases, including cholera and typhoid fever.

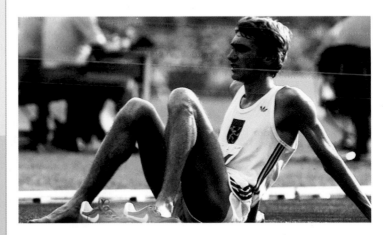

During performance and training, athletes lose a great deal of body fluid through sweating. To avoid dehydration, they need to drink lots of liquids.

SEE ALSO

COFFEE AND TEA • MUSCLE • SKIN • SWEAT

Q & A

Is it safe to drink water directly from a faucet?

In many parts of the world, especially in developing countries, faucet water is not sterilized and may contain bacteria that can cause serious health problems. In the United States, Canada, and many other countries, drinking water is chlorinated, so such health threats are likely to have been eradicated. Other problems may occur if you ingest too much lead from water in old pipes or faucets (faucets made after 1997 contain less lead). If you are in any doubt, you should run the water for one minute before using it, use cold water for cooking, and drink bottled water instead.

I've heard that asbestos can cause some types of cancer. Is there any risk of this from drinking water that has passed through cement-impregnated asbestos pipes?

No. Surveys of areas where these types of pipes have been in use for many years show that there is no increased risk of cancers of the bowel or abdomen.

Elbow

Q & A

I get an odd sensation in my elbow when I bang my funny bone. What causes such a strange feeling in this bone?

One of the nerves of the arm, the ulna nerve, lies in a groove of bone near the tip of the elbow. When the elbow is hit, the nerve becomes pinched in the groove, generating the tingling, painful sensation that gives the funny bone its name.

I injured my right shoulder recently, and now I am having some difficulty moving my right elbow. Why would a shoulder injury affect my elbow?

Many of the elbow's movements depend on the actions of muscles that are attached at one end to the shoulder and at the other end to the bones of the forearm. Because these muscles are involved in elbow movement, any injury to the shoulder can also affect the elbow.

The humerus, ulna, and radius meet at the two joints that form the elbow (1). The biceps muscle runs from the shoulder to the top of the radius; the triceps runs from the shoulder to the humerus and ulna (2).

The elbow is one of the most important joints in the body. Three main bones meet there: the radius and the ulna (which are the two bones of the forearm) and the humerus (which is the single long bone in the upper arm). The elbow is a double joint. The humerus and the ulna (the longer of the forearm bones) are linked with a hinge joint, which enables the arm to bend up and down. The humerus and the radius are linked with a ball-and-socket joint, which enables the arm to be twisted to and fro and the position of the hand to be changed.

The ends of each of the bones in the elbow are covered with a smooth cartilage, which provides a low-friction surface. The elbow joints are lubricated with a clear liquid called synovial fluid. The muscles that control elbow movement are linked to the bones by tough tendons. Bursae, little pouches filled with fluid, lie between the tendons and bones; they also prevent friction.

The most common wear-and-tear injury is bursitis, in which a bursa becomes swollen and inflamed. This problem is usually caused by injury or pressure but may also be due to a bacterial infection. The treatment includes rest or, if the cause is infection, antibiotics. Another common complaint is tendinitis, or inflammation of the tendons. The condition is called tennis elbow when tendons on the outside of the elbow are affected and golfer's elbow when the tendons on the inside are inflamed. Again, rest is the main treatment required.

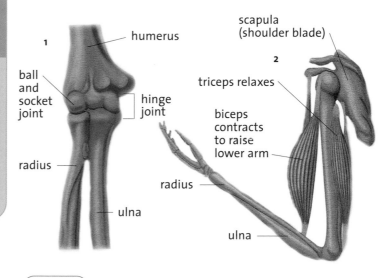

SEE ALSO

FRACTURES AND DISLOCATIONS • JOINTS • LIGAMENTS • SHOULDER • SPORTS INJURIES • TENNIS ELBOW

Exercise

The human body is a living machine, and it needs to exercise to stay in good shape. Regular physical activity works the muscles to keep them strong and boosts the immune system. Exercise keeps the heart and lungs in good working order so these vital organs can better supply the body with oxygen. Regular exercise reduces the risk of heart disease, high blood pressure, insomnia, and diabetes. Exercise also speeds up the metabolism, making the body release fat stores as a source of energy. This increase in metabolism encourages weight loss and helps prevent obesity. There is also the feel-good factor: exercise is known to improve mental health and prevent depression.

Q & A

My mother won't let me go swimming right after I've had a light meal. She says I'll get stomach cramps if I do. Why?

After eating, the stomach and intestines need extra blood to aid digestion. The muscles also need more blood for swimming. If they do not receive enough, they are deprived of oxygen and go into spasms. Therefore, it is best to take a half-hour rest after a light meal so that the stomach can empty itself.

Different types of exercises

Sustained exercise that makes people breathless and sweaty is called aerobic exercise. This form of exercise promotes general physical fitness and a sense of well-being. Aerobic exercise works the heart, lungs, and muscles and increases blood flow through soft tissues. Cycling, running, jogging, swimming, walking, and sports such as rugby and tennis are excellent forms of aerobic exercise. Anaerobic exercise develops muscle strength and power. Weight lifting is perhaps the most familiar form of anaerobic exercise. It involves tensing muscle groups by pulling or pushing against a set of weights. Sprinting is another form of anaerobic exercise that increases short-term muscle strength.

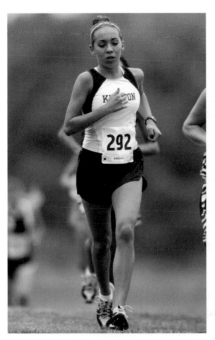

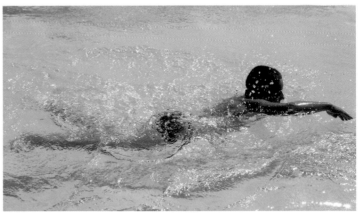

Swimming (above) is an excellent form of aerobic exercise for improving all-around fitness. Because the body is supported in the water, there is less likelihood that soft tissues will be overstrained. Running (left) is a weight-bearing exercise that can help to increase bone strength. Correct techniques should be used, and suitable shoes should be worn, to minimize wear and tear on joints.

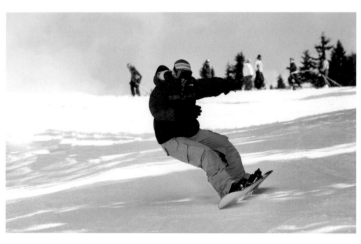

Flexibility exercises are an important part of any exercise program. They improve the range of movement of muscles and joints. Yoga is a good example. It includes exercises to tone muscles, tendons, and ligaments and improve circulation. Yoga includes deep breathing, which helps relax the body and mind.

Vigorous sports, such as snowboarding, force the body to take in extra oxygen. That helps improve the function of the heart and respiratory system.

Amount of exercise

The amount of exercise a person needs to do depends on his or her lifestyle: how active the person is, how much he or she eats and weighs, body metabolism, and so on. Some people are always on the move and stay relatively fit without needing additional exercise. Others sit at a desk all day and get little exercise. It also depends on what a person wants to achieve. Some people simply want to stay healthy, whereas others are training for a particular sport, such as marathon running.

Anyone who is starting a strenuous program of exercise needs to build up stamina and flexibility over a period of time. If a long time has passed since the person did any physical activity, the first few sessions will be uncomfortable and the muscles will ache. However, the body recovers in a week or two, and the benefits soon start to show. Sometimes it is unwise to do any exercise. If people exercise when they are ill—for example, with a cold or influenza—it will simply make them feel more exhausted.

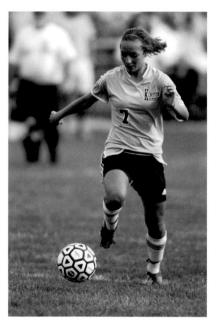

Before high-impact exercise, such as ball sports, people should take time to warm up correctly. Injury is less likely to occur when muscles have been prepared by preliminary stretching exercises.

Response to exercise

People respond to exercise in different ways. Most people feel an increase in endurance following frequent and regular aerobic exercise. However, a few people might double their aerobic capacity, whereas others may not feel much benefit at all. In the same way, only a few people experience significant muscle growth from sustained weight training; most notice only moderate improvements in strength. These differences in response to exercise separate the elite athletes from the rest of the larger population.

Too much exercise

Intense physical activity places enormous stress on the body. Carbohydrates, fats, and proteins are used up to release energy. Tiny tears can form in the muscles and connective tissues. The

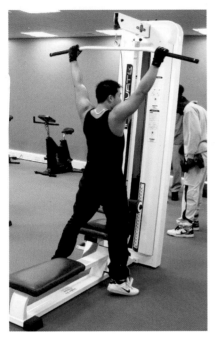

Training with weights builds up muscle size and strength. That type of exercise, which may involve the use of machines, as shown here, or simple hand weights, keeps the muscles in a constant state of tension.

stresses are different for different individuals. However, given enough rest between periods of intense exercise, the body will repair itself and adapt to the training load.

Still, too much exercise is not good for the body. Health experts recommend at least one day of rest between intense exercise sessions to give the body time to recover. In extreme cases, overtraining can lead to circulation problems and fatigue. In addition, sudden bouts of intense exercise can damage muscle tissue. Repeated damage to tissues caused by overexercising may lead to permanent joint problems later on.

Exercise, eating, and obesity

Exercise uses up a lot of energy, so it is essential that people eat a healthy, balanced diet. The food must contain the right balance of carbohydrates, fats, and proteins, as well as vitamins and minerals, to replenish the stocks lost during exercise and aid the recovery process.

Obesity is a serious health problem. Many people take in more energy from food than they use. The body converts the extra energy into fat, which is stored in the body. People then become overweight. In extreme cases, that is called obesity, which substantially increases the risk of serious illness.

Children need to take in lots of energy because their body is growing and developing at a fast rate. However, childhood obesity is becoming more common. It puts children at greater risk of diseases usually seen in adults, such as diabetes, blocked arteries, and high blood pressure. Studies have shown that childhood obesity is much more common if a child's parents are obese. There might be a genetic component to obesity, but it is more likely that family members eat the same fatty foods and avoid physical activity.

Many children get little regular exercise. They spend hours watching television and playing computer games. Health experts recommend that children should do at least one hour of physical activity every day. Young people and children should walk or bicycle to school instead of getting a lift in the car—provided they understand the rules of safety on the highway. A brisk walk is probably the easiest and cheapest form of exercise and can be fitted into the daily routine.

SEE ALSO

AEROBICS • BASAL METABOLISM • FATS • HEART • ISOMETRIC EXERCISES • OBESITY • PHYSICAL FITNESS • REST AND RELAXATION • SPORTS • YOGA

Fainting

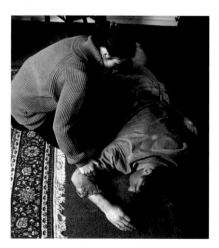

If a person does not recover rapidly from a faint, he or she should be placed in a prone position. This keeps the airway open and lessens the danger of choking.

Fainting, or syncope, usually starts with a sensation of dizziness or light-headedness, followed by sudden loss of consciousness. Someone who is about to faint usually turns extremely pale and his or her skin feels clammy. The person may feel nauseated. Breathing becomes quick and shallow, and as the person faints, he or she may fall to the ground. However, most people recover consciousness in a minute or so.

The most frequent cause of fainting is that not enough blood is reaching the brain. Without the oxygen carried by the blood, the brain cannot work properly. People may faint if their blood pressure is too low to pump enough blood to the brain.

Sometimes, people faint when they stand up suddenly after lying or sitting down. That is because their blood vessels have not adjusted quickly enough to raise the blood as their position changes. Low blood sugar levels (hypoglycemia) can cause fainting. Taking sugar or a sweet drink helps resolve the problem.

Severe emotional stress and mild anemia can also cause fainting. A psychological shock can make the brain act to slow the heart and make it beat less strongly, causing fainting.

Heart valve disease may also cause fainting on exertion. In this case, drug treatment is required and surgery may be considered. Certain poisons and epilepsy can cause blackouts, or fainting. Immediate medical care is needed in the first instance.

First aid for fainting

People who faint regularly should talk to their doctor about the problem. Anyone who remains unconscious for more than a minute or two after fainting needs immediate emergency medical help. If he or she experiences other symptoms, such as numbness or blurred vision, that should also be regarded as a medical emergency.

However, there are a few important rules that can be followed. If someone feels faint, he or she should lie down or sit with the head lowered between the knees so that blood can flow more quickly to the brain. When someone faints, the person should be turned onto his or her side for at least five minutes, and any tight clothing should be loosened. A handkerchief or sponge should be soaked in cold water, wrung out, and put on the person's forehead. When the person recovers consciousness, he or she should be given a few sips of cold water to drink.

SEE ALSO

ANEMIA • BLOOD PRESSURE • CIRCULATORY SYSTEM • DRINKING WATER • HEART • OXYGEN • SKIN • TIREDNESS

Fats

A GUIDE TO
HIGH-FAT FOODS

Foods containing saturated fats

	Percent of fat
Shortening	100
Butter	100
Coconut oil	100
Fried bacon	67
Heavy cream	48
Cheddar cheese	33.5
Broiled steak	32.5
Broiled pork sausages	23
Ground beef	20
Milk	3.6

Foods containing unsaturated fats

	Percent of fat
Olive oil	100
Margarine (vegetable)	100
Peanut butter	48.5
Broiled herring	13
Broiled mackerel	10
Avocado	8

Some foods contain a mixture of saturated and unsaturated fats—for example, mayonnaise is 79 percent mixed fats, and French fries are 20 percent mixed fats, depending on which cooking oil is used.

The fat in the body comes from fats in the food people eat. The digestive system breaks down fats into fatty acids and glycerol. Some fatty acids are broken down at once for immediate energy; if there is any excess, it is stored in the cells under the skin and around the internal organs.

The rate at which the body burns fat is determined by the rate of energy consumption and controlled by hormones from the thyroid gland, the pituitary gland, and the adrenal glands, which secrete adrenaline and noradrenaline. If someone is under stress or getting vigorous exercise, these hormones release more fatty acids into the bloodstream, together with cholesterol. Fatty acids are converted into the body fuel, glucose, in the liver.

Fats provide more energy, weight for weight, than the other two main components of food: carbohydrates and protein. Fats can also make food taste better. The fats in food are of two kinds, called saturated and unsaturated because of their chemical composition. Most saturated fats, such as butter and shortening, come from animals and are solid at room temperature. Unsaturated fats are liquid and come from fish and plants.

Fats and health

Saturated fats have a bad reputation among dietitians because they promote an increase in the tiny transport globules of cholesterol and protein (low-density lipoproteins) that encourage deposition of cholesterol in the arteries. Although cholesterol is vital for making cell membranes, bile, and sex hormones and for maintaining the tissues of the brain, the body can make all it needs in the liver. A high saturated-fat intake interferes with the body's own cholesterol-control machinery, and the bloodstream becomes flooded with cholesterol. Doctors recommend changing from eating high-cholesterol, saturated fats to low-cholesterol, unsaturated fats, particularly polyunsaturates. Onions, garlic, olive oil, and oats are among foods that are thought to help lower the levels of harmful cholesterol.

A diet without any fat would be dangerous, as well as boring and difficult to plan. However, it is perfectly possible to survive on a diet containing only 1 ounce (28 g) of fat a week. A body needs that amount of fat to supply certain fatty acids, which the body is unable to make for itself. Nearly all fats contain these fatty acids; fish, soybeans, and canola oil are good sources.

SEE ALSO

CALORIES • CARBOHYDRATES • CHOLESTEROL • DIET • DIETING • FOOD AND NUTRITION • HEALTH FOODS • OBESITY • PROTEIN

Feet

The feet are mechanical masterpieces. Each foot consists of many small parts—26 bones, 35 joints, and more than 100 ligaments. This structure makes the foot flexible and adapted to walking on uneven surfaces. Most of a foot's power comes from the strong muscles in the leg, helped by a series of small muscles in the foot itself.

The weight of the body is supported on the calcaneus, the largest bone in the foot, which forms the heel, and the heads of the five metatarsals, the long bones that link the toes to the rest of the foot. The bones are arranged in two arches, which provide the strength needed to hold the body's weight.

Fallen arches and foot care

One arch runs across the width of the foot. The other arch runs along the length of the foot and is higher on the inside of the foot than on the outside. If the feet are normal, it is possible to see the difference in the height of this arch from one side to another by making a wet footprint on the bathroom floor. Sometimes, the high side of the arch collapses, because the foot has been strained and its muscles are weakened, causing a flat foot.

The feet have to last for a lifetime and provide support, so people should take good care of them. The feet should be washed at least once a day and dried thoroughly. Socks or pantyhose should be changed every day, and shoes should be aired between wearings. A person's shoes should have plenty of room for the toes. High-heeled shoes put extra strain on the foot muscles, so they should not be worn all the time.

Chilblains and corns

Chilblains are red, swollen areas of soft tissue formed where the skin has been damaged by cold. They may itch and form ulcers. Chilblains are most often found on the toes or the outside of the foot and on the finger joints; they can also form on the ears, nose, and even the calves.

Chilblains are the result of a combination of cold and damp in an area where the blood flow is reduced. Children often get chilblains because they tend to be out in cold weather and may not wear dry shoes or warm gloves. People with poor circulation are

The bones of the feet seen from above and from both sides.

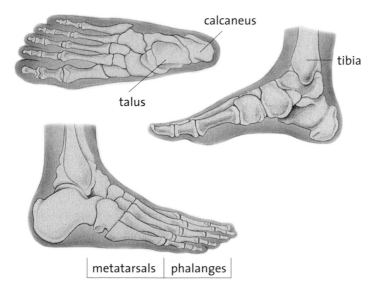

calcaneus

tibia

talus

| metatarsals | phalanges |

COMMON FOOT PROBLEMS

Problem	Cause	Symptoms	Treatment
Athlete's foot	Fungal infection often caught in swimming pools or sports locker rooms, hence its name; aggravated by heavy sweating	Splits in the skin between the toes, often spreading to other parts of the foot	Keep feet dry, especially after washing. Dust with a fungicidal powder or rub in a fungicidal cream. Wear clean socks each day, preferably wool or cotton socks, which absorb sweat.
Bunions	Due entirely to wearing shoes that do not fit properly	Big toe pushed over toward the other toes, causing a deformity of the joint between the big toe and the foot	Correct at an early stage by wearing properly fitting shoes. It is best to consult a podiatrist, who will probably advise exercise to correct the deformity. In extreme cases, surgery may be required.
Chilblains	Contracting blood vessels depriving the skin of oxygen; common in people who are extremely sensitive to cold	Swelling, reddening, itching, and a burning sensation; usually affects the fingers and toes when cold	Prevention is better than cure, so keep the feet warm. Prescribed drugs can improve circulation.
Clubfoot	Generally a congenital defect (present from birth), or caused by an injury that interferes with the foot's natural growth	Foot twisted out of its usual position, with deformed muscles, tendons, and bones	Some conditions can be cured by splinting and manipulation if treated early enough. Special shoes may be required. Severe cases may require surgery.
Corns	Ill-fitting shoes causing pressure points, a buildup of dead tissue, and pain from irritated nerve endings	Painful areas of hard skin on toes, or soft skin between toes	Soaking the foot helps, and corn pads may relieve the pressure. A doctor or podiatrist should be consulted if corns do not respond to simple treatment.
Ingrown toenail	Shoes that do not fit properly	Toenails curving into the flesh; can cause pain, infection, and inflammation	Shoes should be large enough. Nails should be kept short. If there is pain or infection, a doctor or podiatrist should be consulted.
Plantar wart	Infectious wart virus	Painful wart on sole of foot, often covered by a callus	Remove by cauterizing, freezing with dry ice, or surgery.

more likely to get chilblains, as are people who get little or no exercise or whose muscles are wasted by an illness.

Chilblains start as red or purplish blotchy patches that itch and tingle. At this stage, gentle massage and careful warming of the area help. It is important never to scratch these areas. Severe chilblains swell, and tiny blisters containing clear yellow

A flat foot (top right) has no inner arch; the complete sole of the foot touches the ground. The inner arch of the normal foot (bottom right) is higher than the outside one. The arch of a foot helps distribute the body's weight evenly through the heel and toes.

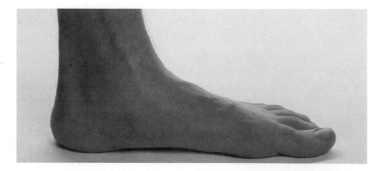

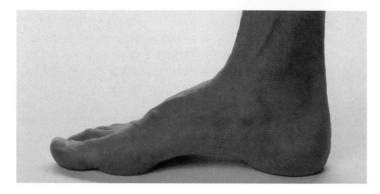

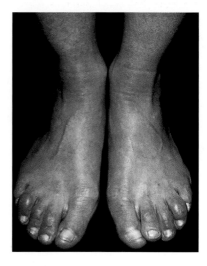

Chilblains are itchy and painful. If precautions are taken in cold weather, chilblains can easily be avoided.

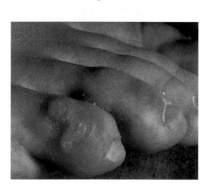

Pressure on the top and side of the little toe, probably from a tight shoe, has caused corns to form there.

fluid may form. In really bad cases, these blisters break down to leave painful ulcer craters. Chilblains usually heal in five to 10 days, but bad cases may take considerably longer. Severe cases need medical treatment. Chilblains can be prevented by wearing warm, loosely fitting clothes in layers and warmly lined waterproof boots or shoes.

Corns, or calluses, are small areas of hard, scaly skin on the toes. They are the result of repeated rubbing or pressure, often from tight shoes. Dead skin cells build up, and the deeper skin cells underneath become inflamed. Corns feel tender under pressure and may ache at the end of the day. Hard corns occur on the tops of the toes; soft corns develop between them.

Corns are treated by rubbing away the excess skin with a pumice stone after a good soaking or by paring off the corn with a special scraper or knife. Corns can also be dissolved with salicylic acid plasters. They are best removed by a doctor or podiatrist.

SEE ALSO

ATHLETE'S FOOT • MUSCLE • SKELETAL SYSTEM • SKIN

Flavonoids

Flavonoids are pigments found in plants. They are present in foods such as fruit and soy products and in tea, red wine, and dark chocolate. There are thousands of different flavonoids with yellow, red, or blue, water-soluble pigments, also known as bioflavonoids or polyphenols. Once thought to be simply the waste products of plants, flavonoids are now known to have important physiological functions and protective qualities.

Studies show that flavonoids can kill some disease-forming microorganisms, relieve inflammation, strengthen capillary walls, prevent blood clots from forming, and modify the actions of many enzymes. Many flavonoids help relieve menstrual and menopausal problems. Flavonoids give some protection against cancers and heart disease.

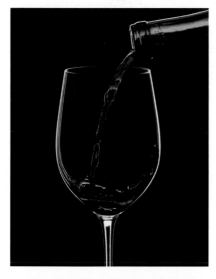

Free radicals

The damage caused to body tissues by poisons, bacterial toxins, smoking, radiation, many disease processes, and other destructive agents arises from the action of chemicals called free radicals. Free radicals attack organic molecules, set up chain reactions in cell membranes and other tissues, and cause widespread molecular damage. To combat these effects, the body synthesizes antioxidants—enzymes that can reverse the effect of harmful free radicals.

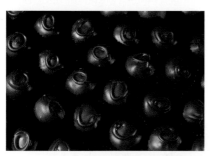

Flavonoids as antioxidants

The principal interest in flavonoids relates to their antioxidant and free radical–scavenging properties. The buildup of cholesterol in artery walls, leading to the development of atherosclerosis, is a major cause of heart attack and stroke. Flavonoids reduce the formation of oxidized low-density lipoproteins (LDLs), which are harmful cholesterol compounds. As a result, flavonoids inhibit the growth of arterial plaque and help prevent blood clotting.

When drunk in moderation, the antioxidant properties of flavonoids in red wine (top) have been found to help prevent the formation of fatty deposits in arteries. The flavonoids in chocolate (bottom) have a similar protective effect.

Flavonoids in wine and chocolate

Antioxidant flavonoids are present in red wine, and many doctors believe that this accounts for the fact that heart attacks are rare in French people, who enjoy a high-cholesterol diet and drink a large amount of red wine. Also, people who eat chocolate regularly seem to be less prone to atherosclerosis. That has been attributed to the flavonoid content of chocolate.

SEE ALSO

ANTIOXIDANTS • CHOLESTEROL • HEART ATTACK • STROKE

Food Additives

The label on any food can, bottle, or package must list all the ingredients. Some of these may be familiar. Others may have strange-sounding chemical names, and some are just vague descriptions such as artificial coloring. However, all of these ingredients have to be approved by the Food and Drug Administration (FDA).

There are several kinds of food additives, including colorings, preservatives, flavorings, texturizers, thickeners, emulsifiers, and supplementary vitamins and minerals, which are added to increase a food's nutritional value.

One reason for clear labeling of foods is that a few people are allergic to some additives. Many of the additives, however, come from natural sources, and many more are closely related chemically to the food products they are found in.

Preservatives

Without preservatives, the vast variety of food on supermarket shelves would not be available all year round. Preservatives are used to stop food from being spoiled by the growth of bacteria and fungi. They also stop food from deteriorating naturally, and they stop oxidation, the process that turns cut apples brown.

Traditional preserving methods such as salting and pickling in vinegar do much the same job as modern preservatives. They are no more natural, however, than modern methods. Salt and vinegar are both chemicals—sodium chloride and acetic acid, respectively. Modern additives such as butylated hydroxyanisole, propionic acid, and sulfur dioxide are closely related to chemicals that are commonly present in food. Vitamin E and vitamin C are health-giving substances that are also used as preservatives.

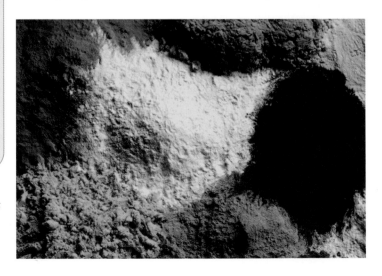

This is a selection of bright food colorings that are routinely added to many foods, including juices and drinks, baked goods, and frozen foods.

Additives are even added to sugar to preserve it and make it taste more palatable to the consumer. Here, the input of additives at a sugar refinery in Florida is being adjusted.

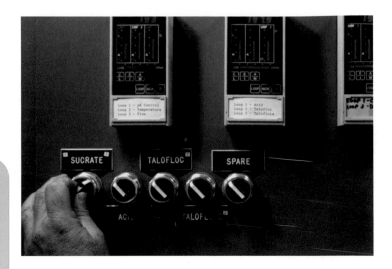

COMMON FOOD ADDITIVES

The following are some of the most common food additives that are listed on cans, jars, and cartons:

Preservatives
• Acetic acid (vinegar)
• Butylated hydroxyanisole (BHA)
• Butylated hydroxytoluene (BTA)
• Citric acid
• Sodium benzoate
• Sodium chloride (salt)
• Vitamin C (ascorbic acid)
• Vitamin E

Thickeners, emulsifiers, and texturizers
• Glycerol monostearate (GMS)
• Lecithin
• Pectin
• Vegetable gums
• Agar
• Carrageen
• Soy
• Gelatin
• Guar gum

Sweeteners
• Saccharin
• Sucrose (sugar)

Flavoring
• Monosodium glutamate (MSG)

Coloring and flavoring

Many foods lose their natural color when they are processed. They look pale and unappetizing. To make food look more appealing, manufacturers add coloring. Some colorings are natural substances, such as chlorophyll.

Flavoring is also added to make food more palatable. Most flavorings are natural extracts that are easily recognized. The substance monosodium glutamate (MSG), which has hardly any flavor itself, has the remarkable property of making meat and fish more flavorful. MSG is often added to Chinese food, although some people react badly to large amounts of this additive, experiencing such symptoms as headaches and chest pains.

Other substances

Texturizers change the consistency of food. Many familiar foods, such as commercial ice cream, would be very difficult to produce without them. Commercial ice cream contains glycerol monostearate (GMS), which makes it creamy, plus gums and alginates (seaweed extracts). Other common texturizers include gelatin (which makes cheesecake smooth) and pectin (which makes jellies set). Added vitamins and minerals rarely increase the nutritional value of foods, except when they are added to replace vitamins and minerals that are lost in food processing, as in milling flour or canning.

SEE ALSO

APPETITE • DIET • FOOD AND NUTRITION • FOOD LABELING • FOOD POISONING • MINERALS • VITAMINS

Food and Nutrition

Foods contain the nutrients that are essential for life. Without food, all living organisms—plants and animals, including humans—eventually die. To grow strong and healthy, people need regular, well-balanced, nutritious meals, and snacks should be healthy ones. Food provides both the materials from which humans make their body tissues and the energy they need to keep alive and active.

Plant and animal food

Plants get their nutrients and water from the soil and the air. They grow with the help of energy from sunlight. Animals use plants and other animals as food. They also need water to drink. The process by which plants and animals take in and make use of their food is known as nutrition. In the last 100 years or so, scientists have discovered a great deal about nutrition. They know which foods people (and plants and animals, too) need to grow strong and to keep healthy. They have found that some diseases are caused by the lack of certain substances in the diet. They have also found that too much of certain foods can cause both short-term and chronic illnesses.

Food choices

Many people do not have much choice about what they eat or even have the option of eating every day. They may live in countries where food supplies are limited or they may not have

Oranges are an important source of dietary fiber and vitamin C.

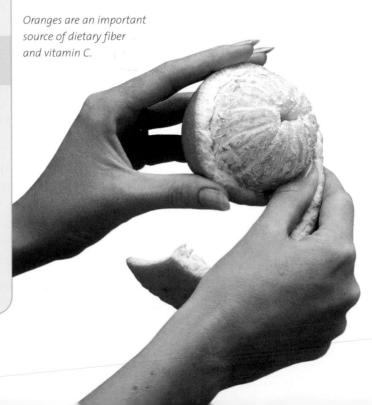

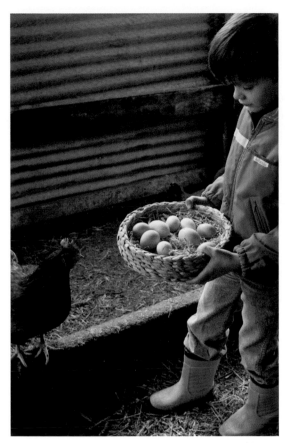

Eggs for breakfast? Until recently, people thought it was healthy to eat an egg a day. Now, some nutritionists believe that people should not eat more than four eggs a week, because eggs contain a substance called cholesterol, which plays a part in diseases of the arteries and heart.

much money to spend on food. Sometimes, they suffer from nutritional diseases. In other countries, such as the United States, there is an immense variety of food available, and people are more likely to suffer diseases of overeating, such as obesity and heart problems. However, more and more people are now interested in eating healthily. If people know about the nutrients the body needs and the foods in which those nutrients are found, they can eat healthily without spending too much money.

Limiting cholesterol

Ideas about the best possible diet are continually changing. For example, there have been many recommendations during the last few years about how many eggs a person can safely eat each week. Opinions vary, but the American Heart Association still recommends no more than four eggs a week.

The association also suggests limiting total cholesterol consumption to 300 milligrams a day. In other words, people should cut down on foods with a high saturated fat content, such as meat, poultry, and dairy products. In addition, it is recommended that everyone should exercise and maintain a healthy body weight.

It is also best to avoid saturated fats present in crackers, cookies, pastries, cakes, doughnuts, french fries, potato chips, and puddings, because these foods are known to increase the bad LDL (low-density lipoprotein) cholesterol in the blood. LDL cholesterol is the type of fat that is deposited in the arteries around the body and causes disease. The good HDL (high-density lipoprotein) picks up loose molecules of cholesterol and returns them to the liver, where they are broken down; they are then eliminated from the body.

Essential nutrients

The nutrients that are essential for life are protein, minerals, fats, carbohydrates, and vitamins. In addition, people need plenty of water. Together, these nutrients will give people

ESSENTIAL NUTRIENTS

Proteins provide the chemical compounds from which all the cells of the body are made. People need proteins to make new tissues and repair old ones. Proteins are also used to make the antibodies that fight infections. They help people digest food and supply them with energy. Proteins are present in animal products, including meat, fish, eggs, and milk, and in some vegetable products, including nuts, peas, beans, and legumes. The body cannot store protein, so it is best to eat some foods containing protein every day.

Fiber is present in vegetable foods. It is made of materials such as cellulose and pectin. Humans cannot digest fiber. It provides no nutrients, but it plays an important part in a healthy diet. Fiber helps move food efficiently through the digestive system. Its bulk stimulates peristalsis, the wave movement that pushes food along the digestive tract. Fiber may also have a helpful effect on the way in which the body uses fats. Studies have shown that people in developing countries whose diet is high in fiber are less likely to develop diseases such as cancer of the colon. Also, people who eat plenty of fiber rarely suffer from constipation. Nutritionists now suggest that everybody should eat a diet high in fiber. Fruits, leafy vegetables, legumes, and unrefined cereals are all high in fiber. Processing removes fiber as well as nutrients.

Carbohydrates, which are present in starchy and sugary foods, are major sources of energy and supply most of a person's calories. Cereals, bread, potatoes, rice, and pasta are high in complex carbohydrates. Simple carbohydrates (sugars) are present in cookies, cakes, and candies. Sugar is high in energy but provides "empty" calories with no vitamins or minerals. Sugar also encourages tooth decay. Extra calories present in starch and sugar are stored as fat.

Fats provide energy and some essential vitamins and acids. They also make food taste pleasant. Fats are present in milk, meat, olives, nuts, and seeds. Excess dietary fat is stored in the body as fatty tissue. Animal fats, and fats from some plants, are saturated fats. Eating too much saturated fat can raise the blood cholesterol level. Unsaturated fat, which is present in fish, chicken, turkey, and most vegetables, is healthier to eat.

Vitamins are chemicals that the body needs to function properly. Vitamin A helps people see well in the dark, and vitamin C keeps the blood vessels healthy. Vitamins C and E are anti-oxidants. Vitamin K helps the blood clot. Vitamins are present in fruits, vegetables, milk, and meat. Methods used for food processing and long storage of food can make supplementation with vitamins necessary. Extra vitamins should be taken only if a doctor recommends them.

Minerals are essential for good health and to keep the body working properly. Iron is needed to carry oxygen around the body in the bloodstream; calcium and phosphorus build strong bones. Each person needs only small amounts, and people eating a sensible daily diet should get enough minerals in their food. Pregnant women may need extra iron but should take mineral supplements only if a doctor advises this. Salt is a mineral; too much salt can be bad, particularly if someone has hypertension (high blood pressure).

Water is essential; it makes up more than half of the body content. It helps in the digestion and absorption of food, carries food to the tissues, and carries away waste products. People can live for weeks without food but would die in a few days without water. The body loses 4 pints (1.9 l) of water daily in urine, feces, perspiration, and the moist air that is breathed out. About 70 percent of food consists of water, but people should also ensure that they drink at least eight cups (1.9 l) of liquid a day, preferably in the form of water rather than other drinks.

the materials for making and repairing body tissues and the energy for carrying out everyday activities.

The energy people get from food is measured in units called calories. If people eat food containing more calories than their body uses, the extra calories are stored in the body as fat. If people eat fewer calories, the body draws on its fat stores for energy and weight is lost. Growing children and people who exercise a lot or do hard physical work use up more calories than people who are inactive. Children and active people need to eat more calories. To stay at the same weight, people need to eat only as many calories as they use.

For many years, scientists have been using the concept of a food pyramid to help people understand about healthy eating. The pyramid shown here was newly designed in 2005 by the United States Department of Agriculture to emphasize the importance of both diet and exercise.

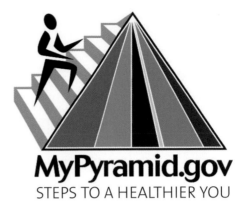

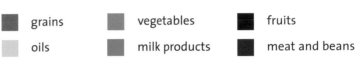

■ grains	■ vegetables	■ fruits
■ oils	■ milk products	■ meat and beans

Food groups

To help people know what they should be eating, scientists have devised a food pyramid that divides foods into different groups, which are represented by six differently colored bands. The different sizes of the bands show the proportion from each food group that should be eaten each day. The wider the band at the base, the more of that food should be eaten. The narrowest band (yellow) represents oils and fats, which should be eaten sparingly. The bands that are widest at the base remind people to eat mostly foods without solid fats and added sugar. The emphasis is on a high-fiber, low-fat diet. Whole grains, fruits, and vegetables are extremely important food items.

This system was designed to help people make healthier food choices. It also reflects the government's new dietary guidelines, including the importance of balancing what people eat with their physical activity; the steps at the side of the pyramid remind people to be active every day.

The orange band represents grains. Everyone should aim to eat 3 ounces (84 g) of whole-grain bread, cereals, rice, or pasta every day. Vegetables are represented by the green band. People should vary their choices and include dark green, leafy, and orange varieties, plus dry beans and peas. Spinach, carrots, and squash provide vitamin A, and many vegetables also provide vitamin C, calcium, iron, and fiber.

The red band indicates fruits, which can be fresh, frozen, canned, or dried. Citrus fruits, tomatoes, strawberries, pineapples, canteloupe, and papaya are rich in vitamin C and also contain

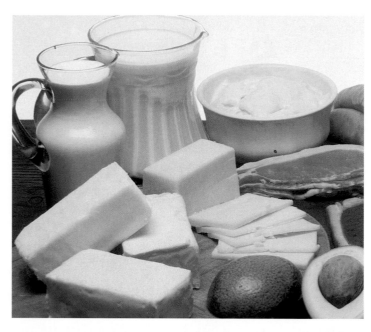

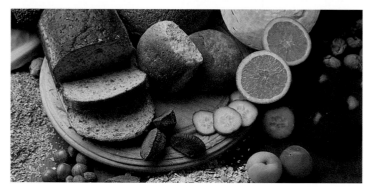

Dairy products (top) such as cream, butter, and cheese are all high in saturated fats. So are bacon, sausages, and red meat. Avocados also contain fat, but it is the healthier, unsaturated type. Whole-wheat bread and fresh fruits (bottom) contain dietary fiber, an important substance that helps keep the body functioning efficiently.

vitamin A, iron, and calcium. Other vegetables and fruits contain vitamins B_1 and B_2, calcium, iron, minerals, carbohydrates, and fiber.

Small amounts of oils or fats (yellow band) should be chosen from fish, nuts, and vegetable oils. Solid fats such as butter, lard, and shortening should be avoided if possible. Milk products (blue band), including cheese, milk, and yogurts, should preferably be fat-free or low-fat—the protein and calcium content is the same, but the fat has been removed.

Meat and beans are protein-rich foods that are represented by the purple band. It is best to choose low-fat or lean meat and poultry and to vary the choices to include more fish, beans, peas, nuts, and seeds.

Harmful fats occur in many foods. Often, they are hidden in cakes and cookies, along with added sugars that do nothing but make people overweight and unhealthy. Everyone should eat as few of these types of foods as possible. It is also better to avoid foods fried in oils or fats, as well as sweets and candies made with butter, sugar, and cream.

Preparing and choosing carefully

The best food ingredients can do little good if they are not properly prepared. An example of this is the way in which rice is polished to remove its husks. Some people think that polished rice tastes better, but removing the husks also removes most of the nutrients. Many people suffer from deficiency diseases that could have been prevented by eating unpolished rice. In a similar way, white flour and its products are often used instead of whole wheat, even though much of the goodness has been removed. In the United States, nutrients are added to white flour to replace those lost in the milling. Nutrients are also added to foods such as milk and margarine to help ensure that people get enough vitamins and minerals.

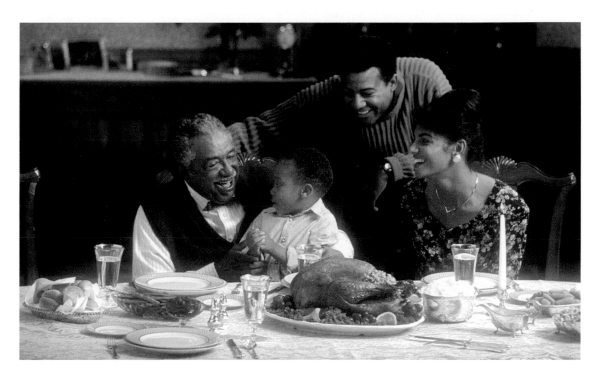

Food should look good as well as taste good, to encourage people to eat. This meal contains a good balance of ingredients. It looks appetizing as well as being healthy.

Cooking food by an appropriate method is an important factor in how beneficial it is. For example, frying depletes nutrients, and vitamins A, B, C, D, E, and K are lost. Vegetables cooked for too long in large amounts of water lose vitamins and minerals.

It is also important that food is grown and prepared in hygienic conditions; otherwise, it may be contaminated with harmful chemicals or disease-causing organisms. Food should always be fresh; fresh or frozen vegetables contain more vitamins than wilted ones.

Changing habits

Making food look and taste good makes it more appetizing and easier to eat. Taste is partly a matter of habit; people like the tastes they are used to. However, tastes can be changed, and because it is now known that eating too much saturated fat, sugar, and salt may be harmful, more cooks are using only small amounts of these substances in their food.

Different foods may taste strange at first, but people soon learn to enjoy the new flavors. Many people now substitute the healthier polyunsaturated fats, such as corn and sunflower oils (and spreads made from them), for butter and shortening.

There are sometimes hidden dangers in food. For example, many processed foods include sugar and salt, and chocolate and candy contain large amounts of fat. Soft drinks are often high in sugar; diet, low-sugar, or reduced-calorie versions are healthier. Food additives, which are substances added to foods to improve their color or flavor, or to preserve them longer, can cause allergic reactions in some people.

As people have become much more conscious of the harm they can do to themselves by not eating sensibly, many have started to change their food habits. Before long, healthy eating may become the norm and people will lead a longer and healthier life.

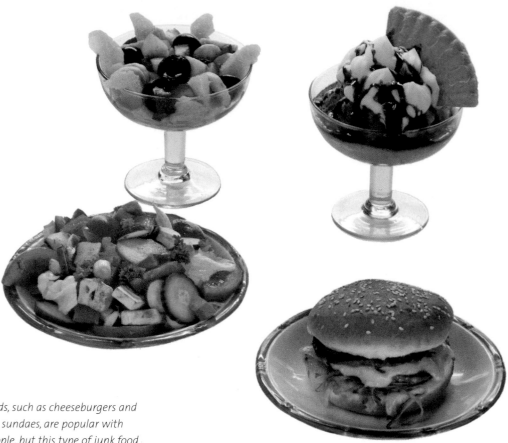

Some foods, such as cheeseburgers and chocolate sundaes, are popular with many people, but this type of junk food contains high levels of sugar and harmful fats. Mixed salad and fresh fruit, properly prepared and presented, are attractive and make far healthier alternatives. Once people get used to eating fresh foods such as these, they may find the taste of junk food less appealing.

> **SEE ALSO**
>
> **ANOREXIA AND BULIMIA • CALORIES • CARBOHYDRATES • CHOLESTEROL • DIET • DIETING • FATS • FOOD ADDITIVES • FOOD LABELING • MINERALS • NUTRITIONAL DISEASES • OBESITY • PROTEIN • SUGARS • VITAMINS • WEIGHT CONTROL**

Food Labeling

The aim of food labels is to provide people with useful information about the food they eat and to help them make better choices. Food labeling follows legal rules set out in 1990 by the Nutrition Labeling and Education Act. These rules were designed by the U.S. Food and Drug Administration (FDA).

By law, all food labels must contain the common name of the food, the name and address of the company that made it, and the amount present (usually by weight). Freshness dates are marked, and labels must list the ingredients in order of content.

The law also requires food labels to provide nutritional data. All the facts are based on one serving, so the first thing the label must identify is the size of one serving. Nutritional facts include the proportions of carbohydrates, fats, and proteins present in the food, as well as any vitamins and minerals. The label must show the energy value of the food, measured in units called calories, as well as how much energy comes from the fat content of the food. Finally, the label must show the recommended daily allowance (RDA) for each nutrient. The RDA is measured as a percentage of an average dietary intake of 2,000 calories each day for women and 2,500 calories each day for men.

Health claims and food additives

The FDA sets standards for the claims food manufacturers use to promote their products. One common example is the term *low fat*. According to the FDA, a food can be labeled as low fat when it contains 3 g or less per serving. Similar definitions exist for many other terms used on food labels.

Substances called food additives improve foods in various ways. Preservatives help food stay fresher for longer, and salt, spices, and sweeteners make food taste better. Dyes improve color; vitamins and minerals add nutritional value. Some additives may cause health problems in people with allergies, so the label must list all additives.

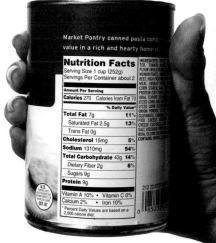

Everything in this can must be listed on the label, together with information such as amount, nutritional data, energy values, and freshness.

SEE ALSO

CALORIES • DIET • DIETING • FATS • FOOD ADDITIVES • FOOD AND NUTRITION • HEALTH FOODS • WEIGHT CONTROL

Food Poisoning

Food poisoning results from eating food contaminated with bacteria or chemicals, or some other poisonous substance. Although the causes vary, the main symptoms are the same: vomiting, pain in the abdomen, and diarrhea, which all begin within a few hours of eating. Most people recover quickly, but the symptoms can be dangerous for children and elderly people. If symptoms are severe, a doctor should be called.

Food is easily contaminated with bacteria unless it is stored and handled hygienically. It is important to wash the hands carefully before touching food or eating and to keep kitchens and utensils clean. People should never prepare food if they have boils or other infections on their hands. Similarly, people should never accept food from a food handler with infected hands.

Infective bacteria in food include salmonella, dysentery, and paratyphoid bacteria. They can come from uncooked or undercooked food or from food that has been cooked when only partially defrosted. Poisons (toxins) can also be produced by bacteria in food, including staphylococcal bacteria and *Clostridium botulinum*. Botulism is a rare but dangerous form of food poisoning that results from eating contaminated, badly preserved food. Anyone with botulism needs immediate hospital treatment, because the infection is life-threatening.

Shellfish living in polluted water are often contaminated, so people should be careful where they get shellfish from. Fruits and vegetables should be washed to rid them of insecticides that have been sprayed on them. Mushrooms or berries should never be eaten unless one is sure that they are not poisonous.

Q & A

My grandmother says that a bit of dirt won't do you any harm. Is she right?

Generally, yes. Household dirt contains millions of micro-organisms; if eaten, most of them are destroyed by the acid in the stomach before they can cause illness. This is why children can eat sand or even worms and come to no harm. Dirt left on food, however, can breed bacteria, which produce toxins that cannot be neutralized by stomach acid. Bacterial toxins can cause food poisoning, such as salmonella and dysentery.

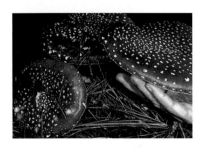

No one should risk even tasting a growing mushroom. Deadly ones can look identical to harmless ones.

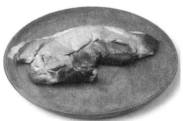

Undercooked meat should never be eaten. Uncooked and cooked meats should never be stored together.

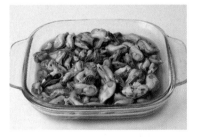

Polluted water can contaminate shellfish. A cooked but unopened mussel must never be eaten.

SEE ALSO

DIGESTIVE SYSTEM DISEASES AND DISORDERS • SALMONELLA

Fractures and Dislocations

A fracture is a break in one of the bones of the body. Some fractures are simple breaks that heal quickly and easily; in other, more serious fractures, the bones may be broken into several pieces. This type of break requires skilled treatment and takes time to heal properly. A dislocation is the displacement of a bone from its socket or from an associated bone.

A simple (closed) fracture is one in which a bone is broken but the skin is intact and the tissues around the break are virtually unharmed. In a compound (open) fracture, the skin is broken by the bone. This type is more serious because there is a much greater risk of infection. When the bone has broken into several pieces, the fracture is described as comminuted. When one end of the broken bone has been driven into another bone, it is an impacted fracture. A depressed fracture is one in which the broken bone is pressing down on the structure underneath. Sometimes, the bone is not broken right through but is simply cracked. Such fractures are known as greenstick fractures. That type of injury is most common in children, whose bones are still growing and are relatively supple.

It takes a great deal of force to break a healthy bone. Fractures are most often caused by accidents such as falls. Elderly people, whose balance is poor, fall more often, and their bones tend to break more easily than those of younger people. Some diseases, including osteoporosis, make the bones so brittle that they break for little or no apparent reason. These types of fractures are known as pathological fractures.

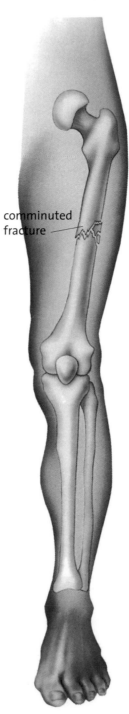

comminuted fracture

In this comminuted fracture of the femur (thighbone), the bone has shattered into small pieces. Treatment involves operating to remove fragments, joining the bone ends with a metal plate, and immobilizing the limb in plaster.

Symptoms and treatment

The most obvious symptom of a broken bone is pain, and damaged tissues in the area around the break may cause the area to swell and look deformed. Movement and pressure may make the pain worse. Broken bones in the hands and feet and broken ribs may be mistaken for sprains or torn muscles, but a limb that is broken cannot be used. The chief danger from a fracture is shock, caused by pain and blood loss. Bone, like any other tissue of the body, has a rich blood supply; the bigger the bone that breaks, the greater the loss of blood. Broken bones may also damage the tissues around them.

Broken bones need medical treatment. A doctor should be called, or the person should be taken to the hospital by ambulance. The victim should be moved as little as possible, particularly if there is any danger of a back injury. When the patient reaches the hospital, he or she will be treated for pain and shock and given an X-ray to assess the damage. The broken bones will then be put in the correct position. A shattered or awkwardly broken bone may need to be repaired with a metal plate screwed along the bone. Some breaks, such as rib fractures, can be left to heal by themselves, but most fractured bones need to be held in position as they heal. This is often done by encasing the area in a plaster cast; a leg may have to be in a cast for 12 weeks or more before it is strong enough to take the body's weight. Bones usually heal extremely well, and in many cases, the fracture leaves no outward sign once it has healed. It may even be difficult to see on a later X-ray.

The supple bones of babies and children may bend and crack rather than break completely. This sort of injury is known as a greenstick fracture (top). The limb should be immobilized in a plaster cast. In a compound fracture (bottom), the broken bone pierces the skin. Damaged tissue and bone fragments must be removed, the bone must be realigned, and the limb must be set in plaster.

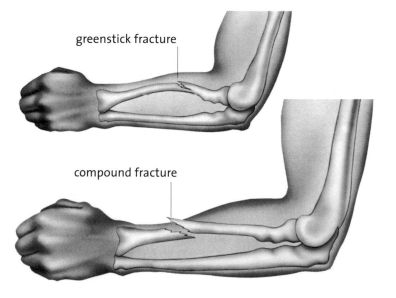

greenstick fracture

compound fracture

The shoulder normally has a rounded contour. If the humerus (armbone) slips out of the scapula (shoulder blade) socket and becomes dislocated, it makes the shoulder take on a square shape (inset).

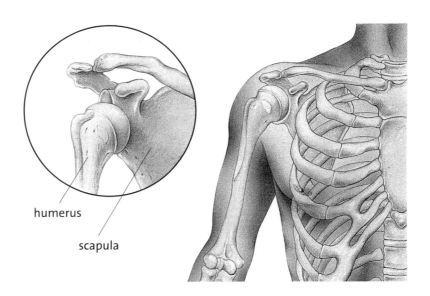

humerus

scapula

Dislocation

Another type of bone injury is a dislocation, in which the bone of a joint is wrenched out of its socket. A dislocated bone is extremely painful because the force of the injury damages the tissues, nerves, and blood vessels around it. The joint swells and needs treatment as quickly as possible. A skilled therapist may be able to put the bone back in position if it is treated immediately, but after 15 minutes or so, the swelling is so great that a general anesthetic is necessary. The shoulders, thumbs, and fingers are the joints most often affected; others include the jaws, elbows, knees, and hips. Some babies are born with dislocation of the hip, which is usually cured by putting the hip in a stabilizing sling for a few months.

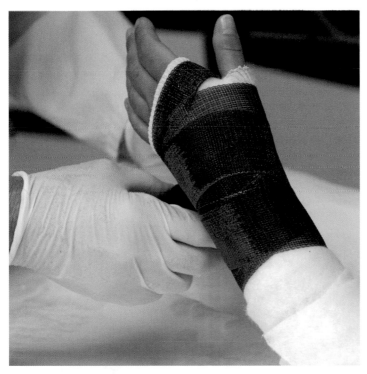

This person has suffered a broken wrist and has had the injury set in a plaster cast that holds together the broken bones to allow them to heal properly.

SEE ALSO

PAIN • SKELETAL SYSTEM • SPORTS INJURIES • SPRAINS AND STRAINS

Glands

Glands are organs that manufacture and secrete substances to perform various functions in the body. There are three main groups of glands: endocrine glands, exocrine glands, and the glands of the lymphatic system. The major endocrine glands—the pituitary, adrenals, thyroid and parathyroid, pancreas, ovaries, and testes—secrete hormones directly into the bloodstream, where they are taken to their target tissues, which are then stimulated into activity. Exocrine glands, such as sweat glands, release a secretion externally, via a canal or duct, to the body's surface. Finally, the lymphatic system produces antibodies and special blood cells called lymphocytes.

The endocrine glands
The body is like a finely tuned musical instrument, with the glands of the endocrine system keeping all the parts working in harmony.

The endocrine system controls many of the vital functions of the body. In turn, the endocrine glands are controlled by a part of the brain called the hypothalamus, which is attached to a master gland called the pituitary, situated at the base of the brain. The pituitary is fed stimulating hormones by the hypothalamus; these hormones act on the other glands in a feedback system. For example, the thyroid gland produces thyroid hormone, which is essential to keep all the body systems active. If the level of thyroid hormone is too low, the pituitary releases thyroid-stimulating hormone to urge the thyroid to produce more of its hormone. Once the level rises, the feedback mechanism ensures that no more stimulating hormone is produced until it is needed. The parathyroid glands are also stimulated by the pituitary to control calcium and phosphorus levels in the blood.

The pituitary gland also controls the release of hormones from organs to ensure that bodily functions are carried out. For example, the pituitary gland stimulates the adrenals to release corticosteroid hormone, which affects metabolism; adrenaline and noradrenaline to increase heart rate and blood flow to muscles; aldosterone to regulate salt excretion; and cortisol to boost sugar levels. The ovaries and testes are stimulated to release male and female sex hormones; and the pancreas, both an endocrine and an exocrine gland, is stimulated to produce two hormones: insulin to regulate blood sugar levels and glucagon to increase blood sugar levels. Apart from its stimulatory function, the pituitary secretes growth hormone; prolactin, to help produce breast milk; a hormone to regulate water balance; and one to contract the uterus (womb) in labor.

Q & A

If glands stop working, is it possible to perform a transplant?

No, but other treatment can be given. If the endocrine glands (which form the hormone system) stop working, a hormone substitute can be given by mouth. If the pancreas stops producing insulin, diabetes results. That is treated with insulin by injection.

I had infectious mononucleosis, and my friend said it was a glandular disease. Was she right?

A common feature of infectious mononucleosis is a swelling of the lymph nodes, and people often refer to this as a swelling of the "glands." However, infectious mononucleosis is a disease that affects the whole body, rather than the lymph nodes alone.

My armpits smell. Is it possible to remove the sweat glands?

Sweat does not smell offensive until it begins to decompose. The solution is frequent washing and using a deodorant. Also, consult your doctor; he or she can recommend other treatments.

FEMALE GLANDS

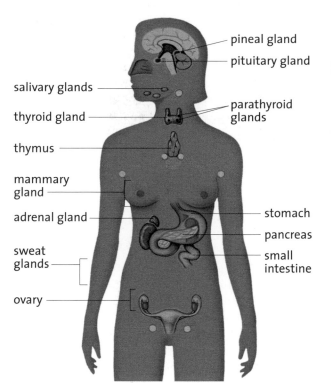

- pineal gland
- pituitary gland
- salivary glands
- thyroid gland
- thymus
- mammary gland
- adrenal gland
- sweat glands
- ovary
- parathyroid glands
- stomach
- pancreas
- small intestine

MALE GLANDS

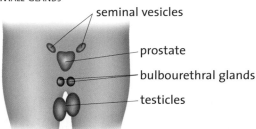

- seminal vesicles
- prostate
- bulbourethral glands
- testicles

This diagram shows the location of the endocrine and exocrine glands in a woman. The yellow spots indicate lymph nodes, which are known as glands but are part of the immune system, along with the thymus. The pineal gland controls body rhythms such as waking and sleeping. A man's glands are the same, except for the reproductive glands (above right). Whereas a woman has mammary glands and ovaries, a man has testicles (which produce testosterone), seminal vesicles, bulbourethral glands, and a prostate gland (which produces seminal fluid).

The exocrine glands

The exocrine glands release secretions to the surface of the body. For example, sweat glands produce sweat, secreted through pores in the skin. Modified sweat glands in the ears produce earwax. Sebaceous glands in the skin produce sebum, which keeps the skin supple. Tear glands produce fluid to lubricate the eyes, and mammary glands produce milk. Other exocrine glands produce digestive fluids. These glands include the salivary glands, the pancreas, glands in the lining of the stomach and the intestines, and the liver.

The lymph nodes

The lymph nodes, which are commonly, but incorrectly, referred to as glands, are part of the lymphatic system. This system is a network of lymph vessels and lymph nodes. The lymph nodes contain lymphocytes, which are blood cells called white cells that help fight the spread of infection. Lymph nodes vary in size from microscopic to 1 inch (2.5 cm) in diameter.

The pineal gland

Deep within the brain, the pineal gland secretes the hormone melatonin, which affects the regulation of the day-night internal body clock. This hormone is secreted mainly during the hours of darkness and is not produced when bright light enters the eyes. If given as a drug, melatonin alters the body clock settings, so it is sometimes taken to prevent jet lag.

> **SEE ALSO**
> BODY SYSTEMS • CALCIUM • DIGESTIVE SYSTEM • GROWTH • SALT • SKIN • SUGARS • SWEAT

Growth

From the time an egg is fertilized to the birth of a baby takes just nine months. This is the most rapid stage of all in the body's growth and development, but a newborn baby is still tiny and helpless. It takes approximately 9 to 10 years before a child is physically capable of being independent, and even longer before mental development is complete.

Infancy

At first, a newborn baby can do little more than suck, swallow, and grasp. During the first year of life, however, the body grows extremely quickly. Nerves develop their interconnections, and as they develop, babies are able to learn to control their movements and to make sense of their surroundings.

After the first year, physical growth slows down and the toddler enters a steadier period of growth, during which more intricate skills are mastered. Each stage in learning, including walking, talking, and reading, depends on the development of the brain and nervous system.

When a baby's bones are first formed, they are made of a flexible tissue called cartilage. As the limbs grow, the cartilage is replaced by fibrous tissue, which gradually solidifies into hard bone, a process known as ossification. At birth, much of the skeleton is still cartilage, and the bones of the skull have not yet joined together; instead, they are flexible, to allow the baby to pass quite easily through the mother's narrow birth canal.

Childhood

All through childhood, and until the body is fully grown, new cartilage cells are made to increase the size of the bones. The bones become longer, thicker, and harder, until they stop growing completely by the mid-20s. At the same time, all the other cells in the body are increasing in number and growing larger.

From about age three until adolescence, children grow approximately 2 to 3 inches (5–7.5 cm) a year. As children grow, the proportions of their bodies change as parts develop

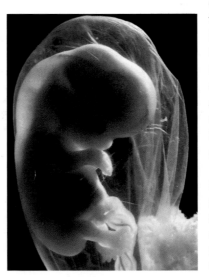

A nine-week-old fetus is just 0.9 inch (2.3 cm) long. All the body parts are present, although they are not fully formed. By the end of pregnancy, the 40-week-old fetus will have fully grown to about 20 inches (51 cm) in length.

at different rates. For example, a baby's head is much larger in proportion to its body than an adult's; its head, therefore, will grow less than the rest of its body.

Adolescence

Throughout childhood, girls are on average around 0.5 inch (1.3 cm) shorter than boys. At about 11, however, girls undergo a sudden increase in height, known as the adolescent growth spurt. They may grow taller than boys of the same age, who start this spurt about two years later. Everything grows during this time—bones, muscles, and organs such as the heart.

Many children change in appearance as the shape of their face changes. The forehead, nose, and chin become less rounded as fat disappears from the face. Boys broaden at the shoulders and girls widen at the hips. The secondary sexual characteristics develop in both girls and boys. Often, this growth is uneven, with muscles growing more slowly than bones, so that adolescents look gangling and out of proportion. In the late teens, growth slows down, and by the early 20s, the body is fully developed.

Variations in growth

Growth is controlled by various hormones produced by the body, including growth hormone, thyroid hormone, and sex hormones. If too much or too little of these hormones is produced, growth will be affected. Children's growth should be checked regularly by a doctor. If they are not developing normally, it may be possible to treat them with the appropriate hormone. Some diseases, and a diet that lacks certain nutrients, may also hinder growth.

Many parents and children worry about the rate of growth during childhood. It is important to remember that this rate varies considerably. Two normal, healthy children who are age seven may differ by as much as 8 inches (20 cm) in height. Girls may begin their growth spurt anytime between 9.5 and 14.5 years; boys may begin their growth spurt between 10.5 and 16 years.

Understandably, those children who start growing late may worry that something is wrong, but there is usually no problem. It is sensible to see a doctor, however, because in most cases he or she will be able to give the necessary reassurance.

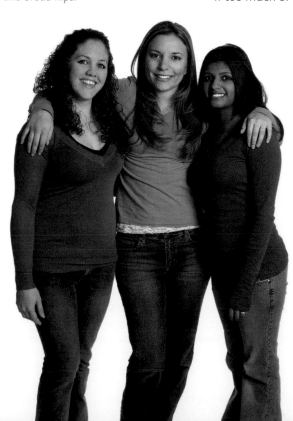

These teenage girls have had their growth spurt. Between the ages of 9.5 and 14.5 years, girls suddenly become much taller, the shape of the face changes, and they develop secondary sexual characteristics, such as breasts and broad hips.

Hormones

A person's rate of growth is controlled by various hormones, two of which are particularly important: growth hormone and thyroxine. Growth hormone is produced by the pituitary gland and thyroxine by the thyroid gland, which lies at the base of the neck. If someone's body is not producing enough of these hormones, growth will be slowed down, although the body remains in proportion. Giving the person additional hormones may allow him or her to develop normally.

Gigantism

If a child grows much taller than normal, he or she may be suffering from a condition known as gigantism. This disorder is caused by an overproduction of growth hormone by the pituitary gland, a pea-size endocrine gland situated in the brain.

Although it is usually possible to stop the extra growth, people with the disorder have been known to reach 8 to 9 feet (2.4–2.7 m) in height. They are generally in proportion, although they usually have extremely large hands and feet.

In some cases, the excess of growth hormone begins after the long bones of the body have stopped growing, in the mid-teens. Then, the hormone causes a disorder known as acromegaly. The bones of the face, jaws, hands, and feet slowly thicken, and the soft tissues of the face, ears, and nose grow thicker, too.

Excess growth hormone is usually caused by a tumor in the pituitary gland. The tumor can be removed by surgery or destroyed by radiation. If the pituitary gland is destroyed by the tumor, the patient will be given replacement hormones.

Dwarfism

People who are unusually short in height, although generally normal in other ways, have traditionally been called dwarfs. Since the term may be hurtful to a person of short stature, thoughtful people now avoid this terminology.

A person's height is ruled by the length to which the long bones in the body finally grow. A condition called achondroplasia prevents these bones from developing normally. People with this inherited condition have a normal-size body, with a rather large head, and legs and arms that are only half the length of normal limbs. They seldom grow to more than 4 feet (1.2 m) in height.

SEE ALSO

BODY SYSTEMS • DIET • FOOD AND NUTRITION • GLANDS • PUBERTY • SKELETAL SYSTEM

Hamstring Injuries

The hamstring muscles are a group of three muscles that form the back of the thigh (the ham area) and span the femur (thighbone). They help bend the leg at the knee and twist the leg in and out.

Hamstring injuries are common, especially among athletes, but they are not serious. The hamstrings are a group of three muscles at the back of each thigh. Individually, they help twist the leg in or out by rotating the knee. Together, the hamstring muscles help bend the leg at the knee. These muscles are long, thin, and easily damaged. A hamstring may tear or become bruised following a blow. Overstretched muscles can also tear when they are tired or are used without being warmed up. The signs of a hamstring injury range from a dull ache to a sharp shooting pain in the back of the thigh. Eventually, the muscle goes into spasm. Ruptured blood vessels can also cause swelling and tenderness in the muscle.

Prevention and treatment

The best way to avoid hamstring injuries is to warm up before exercise by stretching the muscles. Fatigue increases the risk of hamstring injuries, so it is also important to stop before getting too tired. At the first sign of pain, the area should be massaged, and the warm-up exercises should be repeated. A support bandage may be necessary. If the pain continues, all activity should be stopped and medical help should be sought.

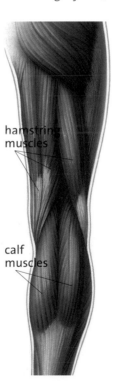

hamstring muscles

calf muscles

If a person suffers such an injury, he or she should stop immediately. It may be tempting to continue, but that only makes the damage worse. The first thing to do is raise the leg and apply a compression bandage to stop any bleeding. An ice pack reduces swelling and inflammation.

Follow-up treatments include ultrasound massage to aid recovery. Heat and conventional massage help disperse blood clots and prevent internal scarring. Stretching exercises also help the muscle recover. Severe hamstring injuries usually require pain relief. Crutches may also be needed to assist walking. Hamstring injuries can take several days to several months to heal.

SEE ALSO

BRUISES • CRAMPS • LEG • LIGAMENTS • MASSAGE • MUSCLE • PHYSICAL THERAPY • SPORTS INJURIES • SPRAINS AND STRAINS

Health Foods

Health foods, also known as whole foods or organic foods, are grown and prepared in a more natural way than commercially processed food. They can be bought in health-food stores or in supermarkets but are often expensive because they are not mass-produced. Most food is treated in some way to make it last longer or look more appetizing. White bread, for example, is made from refined flour; the wheat germ and husk (bran), containing vitamins, minerals, and other health-giving substances, are removed during processing. Coloring, artificial flavoring, and preserving agents are often added to food. Fruits and vegetables are treated with pesticides and chemicals to help produce a maximum-yield crop from each plot of land. These food additives and refining processes destroy much of food's natural goodness. Experts believe that some of these treatments can be harmful to long-term health. Heart disease and some types of cancer, for example, are linked with the consumption of too many refined and treated foods. People are now buying more organic foods than ever before, because of the link with good health.

Health foods retain as much natural goodness as possible. Whole-wheat bread, cereals, and flours contain the wheat germ and husk. Vegetable oils that are polyunsaturated, such as wheat germ, corn, and sunflower oils, are known to be more healthful than saturated fats, such as butter or cream. Health-food stores sell these oils unrefined, so they retain their nutrients, color, and flavor. Free-range eggs are preferable, because the hens are able to run freely outdoors, eating different foods. These scraps provide vitamins and minerals that are not usually present in eggs from caged hens. Fruits and vegetables available in health-food stores are organically grown; manure or compost is used in the soil instead of artificial fertilizers, and pesticides are not used.

husk (provides bran fiber, minerals, and B vitamins)

endosperm (mostly starch and protein, used in white flour)

germ (provides vitamin E and B vitamins)

Whole-grain flour contains vitamins and minerals, much of which is removed from white flour during processing.

Heart

Can healthy people strain the heart through exercise in the same way that they can pull a muscle?

No. In a healthy person, this problem would not happen. However, before people go for a long run, they should remember that "healthy" is not the same as "normal." Coronary artery disease is common and may limit the work the heart can do. People in their forties and fifties are likely to have some degree of artery disease, and it is not unknown in younger people. Everyone should build up to exertion gently to avoid putting the heart under undue stress. People should also do warm-up exercises before they start.

When I get a shock, my heart feels as if it will jump out of my chest. What causes this feeling? Is it serious?

Do not worry; your heart is quite normal. The shock makes your adrenal glands pump out adrenaline, which suddenly drives your heart to beat very fast and forcefully, causing these symptoms.

The heart is a large, muscular organ situated just above the diaphragm in the middle of the chest, although slightly more of it lies on the left side of the body than on the right. The heart's function is to pump blood around two separate circulations, or systems of blood vessels, in the body.

The body's major circulatory system is called the systemic circulation. It is a massive branching network of blood vessels—arteries, veins, and capillaries—to every part of the body and back to the heart. The heart pumps fresh blood filled with oxygen into the aorta, the central artery of the body. From there, the blood is distributed to the rest of the arteries. This blood circulates through the organs and tissues of the body, delivering nutrients and oxygen to them. When all the oxygen has been absorbed from it, the blood is described as deoxygenated. This blood returns to the heart through the veins.

The heart then pumps the deoxygenated blood through its second circuit: this time a short journey to the lungs. This is called the pulmonary circulation, from the Latin word meaning "lung." The lungs replace the used oxygen in the blood and remove the carbon dioxide that has accumulated in it. This oxygenated blood returns to the heart, and the circuit continues.

Structure and working of the heart

The pumping action of the heart is carried out by two pairs of chambers (compartments): the left and right atria (which are the upper chambers) and the left and right ventricles (which lie below the atria). Each chamber is a muscular bag, with a strong, muscular wall called the septum that divides the left and right sides of the heart. The muscular walls of the chambers contract to push the blood along, and valves between the chambers control the direction of the blood flow.

The heart powers both the pulmonary and the systemic circulations in the following way. Blood flows through pulmonary veins from the lungs into the left atrium of the heart. This blood is rich in oxygen, provided by the lungs. The left atrium contracts and pushes the blood into the left ventricle. A valve between the left atrium and left ventricle ensures that the blood cannot flow back the other way. The left ventricle then contracts and pushes the blood out through another one-way valve into the aorta, and this major artery carries fresh, oxygenated blood to all parts of the body. On its return, the used blood has now lost its oxygen and flows into the right atrium of the heart, which pushes the blood into the right ventricle. The right ventricle pumps this blood back to the lungs to pick up more oxygen, thus completing the double circulation. One-way valves ensure that the blood flows one way only. With each heartbeat, the two atria contract, followed by the two ventricles. When the body is at rest, this process is repeated between 50 and 80 times a minute.

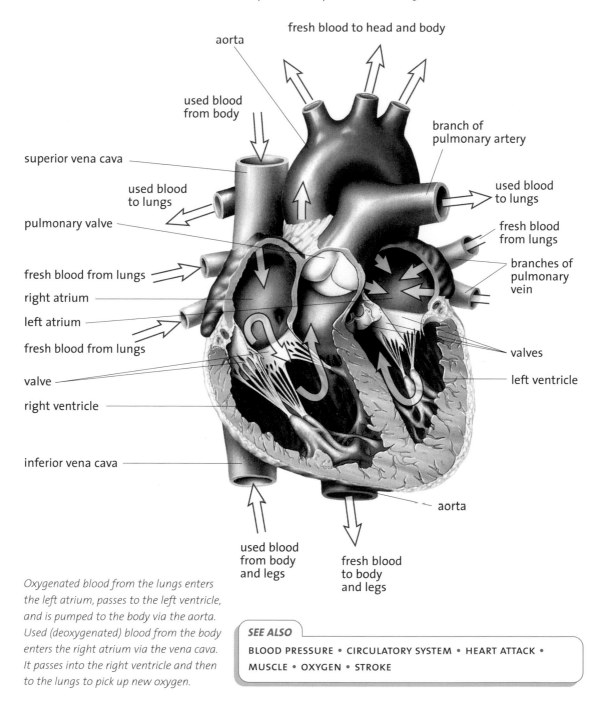

fresh blood to head and body

aorta

used blood from body

branch of pulmonary artery

superior vena cava

used blood to lungs

used blood to lungs

pulmonary valve

fresh blood from lungs

fresh blood from lungs

branches of pulmonary vein

right atrium

left atrium

fresh blood from lungs

valves

valve

left ventricle

right ventricle

inferior vena cava

aorta

used blood from body and legs

fresh blood to body and legs

Oxygenated blood from the lungs enters the left atrium, passes to the left ventricle, and is pumped to the body via the aorta. Used (deoxygenated) blood from the body enters the right atrium via the vena cava. It passes into the right ventricle and then to the lungs to pick up new oxygen.

SEE ALSO

BLOOD PRESSURE • CIRCULATORY SYSTEM • HEART ATTACK • MUSCLE • OXYGEN • STROKE

Heart Attack

A heart attack occurs when the blood supply to the heart is obstructed. The coronary arteries are vessels that supply the heart with blood rich in food and oxygen. Heart attacks occur when these arteries become clogged with fatty deposits, a condition known as atherosclerosis. Blood clots can form around the deposits and block the artery. In turn, that obstruction blocks the blood supply to the heart. The person will then feel the chest pain that indicates a heart attack.

Warning signs

A heart attack may come as a surprise, but most people get a warning. When the coronary arteries start to get blocked, the heart works harder during exercise or excitement. That may cause a crushing, suffocating pain in the chest, which may spread to the arms and neck. Anyone who experiences this pain, called angina, should consult a doctor immediately. Smokers, diabetics, and those with a family history of heart attacks are most at risk.

Often, the main symptom of a heart attack is a severe pain in the chest. The pain is usually more acute than angina; it may be so severe that the person collapses.

In some cases, there is little pain and the person may mistake the heart attack for indigestion or heartburn. Other symptoms include sweating, shortness of breath, and a weak or slow pulse.

Diagnosis and treatment

A heart attack is a life-threatening condition. It requires immediate hospital treatment. In the hospital, doctors confirm the heart attack with blood tests. An electrocardiogram (ECG) may be given to monitor the electrical activity of the heart. In this procedure, the heart's tiny electric currents are recorded on a machine called an electrocardiograph, which prints out the result—the ECG—on a roll of paper. Any heart disorder, such as a heart attack, shows up as a change of pattern.

Morphine is usually given as pain relief. More drugs may be given to improve the circulation and limit damage to the heart muscle. If there are no complications, most patients can return home to rest after a week or so.

Q & A

Is there anything I can do now to prevent a heart attack from occurring in later life?

Do not smoke. Smoking significantly accelerates the pace of atherosclerosis (the hardening and thickening of the artery walls), which is the cause of coronary artery disease, and it is thus a main factor in heart attacks. There is also strong evidence that if you eat less food that contains saturated fats (which are mostly of animal origin, such as butter and cream), you can reduce the risk that your coronary arteries will become narrowed by cholesterol deposits. Aerobic exercise in the form of running, cycling, and swimming may also help.

My father, who has always led an extremely active life, has just had a heart attack. Does this mean that he will have to slow down now?

Not necessarily, unless he has been told to do so by his doctor. Your father should avoid sudden bursts of activity, however, and build up to any exertion more gradually than he did before.

SEE ALSO

BLOOD PRESSURE • CIRCULATORY SYSTEM • HEART • OXYGEN • PAIN • STROKE

Heat Sickness

Q & A

What is the difference between sunstroke and heatstroke?

There is no difference. Both terms describe the serious and potentially fatal condition that can occur if the body is excessively heated, resulting in the total breakdown of the temperature-regulating mechanism in the body. Heatstroke is a more accurate name, because you can suffer from its effects away from the sun. If the temperature is high enough, you can get heatstroke even when not in direct sun.

The body temperature is normally about 98.4°F (37°C). If the surrounding temperature rises, the body's thermoregulation system reacts: it stops the body from overheating and protects the brain, which cannot tolerate high temperatures. The body reacts in two ways. Its main reaction is to perspire. As the sweat evaporates, the skin cools. The body can also lose heat by the dilation of blood vessels; when they widen, more blood reaches the skin, which takes on a flushed appearance, and the blood cools. Sometimes, the body is badly affected by heat. Heat cramps, which are caused by physical effort in extremely hot conditions, are an occupational hazard of miners and firefighters.

In the condition called heat exhaustion, or heat prostration, victims may collapse as a result of excessive loss of fluid and salt. Victims sweat so much that their body temperature remains normal. In very hot, damp places, however, the sweat may not evaporate and cool the body. Heatstroke—or sunstroke—may occur; in this condition the patient's temperature rises rapidly. This is a very serious condition that can lead to permanent brain damage and even death. People who move from a cool climate to a hot one are at risk of heat exhaustion or heatstroke. Outdoors, they should wear light clothes and a sun hat and should be careful not to sunbathe or exercise for too long. A lot of fluid is lost during perspiration; this fluid has to be replaced by taking extra liquids and salt. Anyone who shows signs of heat sickness should be taken to a cool place as soon as possible and given salty water to drink.

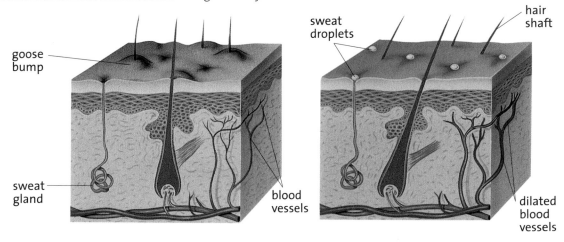

goose bump • sweat gland • blood vessels • sweat droplets • hair shaft • dilated blood vessels

When the body is cold (left), the blood vessels narrow, less sweat is produced, the hair stands straight out from the skin, and goose bumps develop. When the skin is heated (right), the blood vessels dilate, the sweat glands work harder, and the hair lies closer to the skin.

SEE ALSO

DRINKING WATER • EXERCISE • SALT • SKIN • SUNBURN • SWEAT

Hernia

A hernia is a bulge of soft tissue that forces its way through an opening or weak place in the surrounding muscles and fibrous connective tissues. If it is an external hernia, the bulge of tissue is covered with a layer of fat and skin. The bulge usually contains either a loop of small intestine or part of the fatty membrane that covers the intestines. Hernias most often appear in the abdomen. A hiatal hernia, for example, is formed when part of the stomach pushes up into the chest through a weak place in the diaphragm. Other hernias may occur in the groin (inguinal or femoral hernia) and near the navel (umbilical hernia). Hernias may be caused by straining the muscles while doing heavy work or by allowing muscles to become weak through lack of exercise.

Symptoms and treatment

Some hernias produce no symptoms, but those near the surface of the abdomen may cause a tender lump, which disappears temporarily when pressed. A hiatal hernia may allow food and acid to move from the stomach back into the gullet. That causes a burning pain behind the breastbone. Sometimes, the blood supply to the hernia may be totally cut off. When this happens, the tissues within the bulge swell, die, and decay. This condition is known as a strangulated or incarcerated hernia. It is extremely painful and needs an immediate operation.

Most hernias need to be treated by surgery. The bulging tissue is pushed back into place and the defect repaired. This is usually a fairly simple surgical procedure carried out in a hospital. The symptoms of a hiatal hernia can be eased by losing excess weight, taking antacids, and eating small, frequent meals.

Q & A

Don't hernias hurt? My uncle has a hernia, but he says he's not in pain.

Hernias do not usually hurt, except when they first occur—for example, during heavy lifting. Afterward, they may be a bit uncomfortable, but they are usually not painful. If a hernia does hurt, it may be strangulating because its blood supply is cut off; medical advice should be sought.

Can a tendency toward hernias run in families?

Yes, but there is no definite hereditary link. Members of some families tend to do the same types of jobs—for example, those involving heavy labor, which are more likely to cause a hernia.

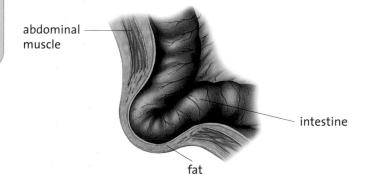

abdominal muscle

intestine

fat

Groin or inguinal hernias are extremely common. They occur more often in men than in women. The soft lump bulges when the patient coughs but disappears when he lies down. This type of hernia can be treated by wearing a truss or by a simple surgical operation.

SEE ALSO

DIGESTIVE SYSTEM • DIGESTIVE SYSTEM DISEASES AND DISORDERS • MUSCLE • RESPIRATORY SYSTEM

Hip

The hips are the largest and strongest joints in the body. They carry all the body's weight and enable a person to stand, walk, and run. A hip joint is literally a ball-and-socket joint. The ball of the joint is a projection on the end of the femur (the thighbone). It fits into the socket, which is a cup-shaped hollow in the iliac bone. The iliac bone is part of the pelvis.

The hip joint is padded with cartilage and fatty tissue and lubricated by a special fluid. Tough ligaments hold the joint in position and prevent the ball from slipping out of the socket. Muscles lying over the ligaments enable people to move their legs in many different positions.

In some newborn babies, the hips slip out of joint easily. This problem requires immediate treatment. In some elderly people, the joint may wear out. It can usually be replaced by an artificial joint made of stainless steel and plastic.

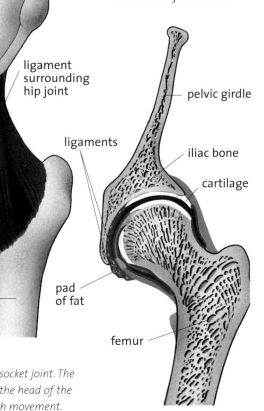

pelvic girdle

ligament surrounding hip joint

ligaments

pad of fat

femur (thighbone)

pelvic girdle

iliac bone

cartilage

femur

The hip is a ball-and-socket joint. The cartilage that covers the head of the femur ensures smooth movement. The joint is lubricated by special fluid produced by membranes. Ligaments hold the hip in position, and pads of fat help cushion the joint, acting as shock absorbers.

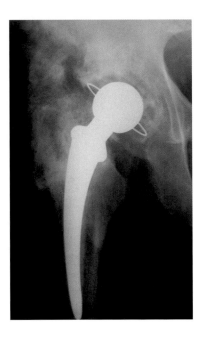

An artificial hip can replace a badly fractured one. This artificial hip (above) is made of stainless steel and titanium.

SEE ALSO

FRACTURES AND DISLOCATIONS • JOINT DISORDERS • JOINT REPLACEMENT • JOINTS • LEG • LIGAMENTS • SKELETAL SYSTEM

Homeostasis

Homeostasis is the mechanism that keeps a body's systems stable and in balance. The human body is a complex machine with many control systems that keep it running smoothly. The body works best if its internal conditions are kept more or less the same all the time. The way the body keeps things the same is called homeostasis, meaning "same" and "still." Homeostasis helps maintain the right amount of water or salts in the body, keeps the body at a certain temperature, and makes sure that the body is operating at the correct rate for whatever a person is doing at any one time.

Homeostasis in action

Since homeostasis happens automatically, people do not have to think about it, but they can still see when it is happening. For example, when a person exercises strenuously, the muscles powering the legs and arms produce heat. This heat increases the body temperature. If that process was allowed to continue, it would soon get too hot for the body to function properly. Detectors throughout the body sense the temperature increase and tell the homeostatic system to cool down the body.

These homeostatic messages are sent around the body via the network of nerves and by chemical messengers called hormones. Nerve signals make sweat glands pump water onto the skin to cool the surface of the body. Other glands produce hormones, which make the blood vessels in the skin expand, so the skin becomes red as it fills with blood. That helps heat in the blood escape from the body. When the body is cold, however, blood vessels in the skin constrict (become narrower), making the skin pale as blood moves into the middle of the body, and heat is prevented from being lost to the outside.

Negative feedback

Homeostasis works by the principle of negative feedback: If one condition changes, a negative-feedback system works to bring that condition back to how it was before the change took place. For example, if the amount of water in the body gets too low, a negative-feedback system operates to increase the water level by making the person feel thirsty, so that he or she will drink some water. If the water level gets too high, negative feedback reduces the level by making the person urinate.

Q & A

I've heard that hunger is part of a homeostatic mechanism. Is that true?

Yes. Hunger is induced when brain cells detect low levels of blood sugar (glucose) and emptiness in the stomach. The sensation of hunger prompts the individual to seek and eat food. If this is successful, the blood sugar rises and the stretch receptors in the stomach signal that no more food is currently required.

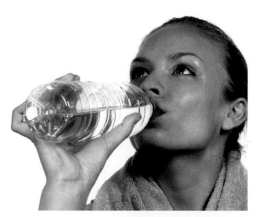

Feeling thirsty is an example of homeostasis in action; the body's mechanisms have detected that the level of water is too low, and a negative-feedback system initiates thirst.

SEE ALSO

BODY SYSTEMS • DRINKING WATER • EXERCISE • GLANDS • NERVOUS SYSTEM • SALT • SWEAT

Hyperventilation

Hyperventilation is a syndrome (a collection of symptoms) usually caused by anxiety. It may also occur during panic attacks. Anxious people sometimes feel as though they cannot get enough air into their lungs. As a result, they breathe too rapidly and deeply, lowering the level of carbon dioxide in the blood. Consequently, they feel dizzy and have numb and tingling hands and feet. Their fingers and toes may also go into a painful and uncontrollable spasm.

Some people hyperventilate if they experience pain. The quickest cure is for the patient to breathe into a small paper bag for a few minutes. The carbon dioxide breathed out is then breathed back into the lungs. Once people realize that they have been hyperventilating, the problem usually stops.

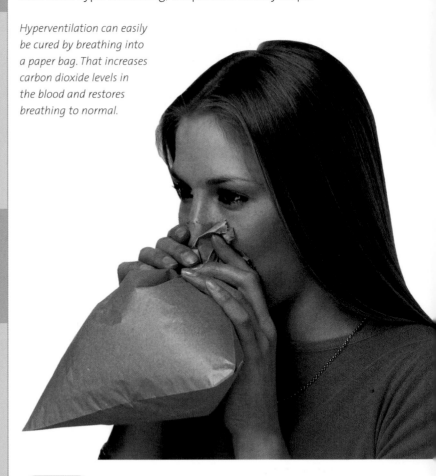

Hyperventilation can easily be cured by breathing into a paper bag. That increases carbon dioxide levels in the blood and restores breathing to normal.

Q & A

Once, after I received some bad news, I noticed that I was breathing quickly and had a tingling sensation around my mouth. What caused this?

Hyperventilation, or fast breathing, occurs in some people when they are upset. Hyperventilation causes an abnormal loss of carbon dioxide, a change in blood acidity, and a consequent drop in blood calcium. Nerves require calcium ion movement for proper function, and this is why your nerves were affected.

I'm a little nervous, and I find that I get breathless sometimes. When this happens my fingers start to tingle, and once my hand cramped. What causes these problems?

You have a complaint that is common among nervous people. It is called hyperventilation tetany and is harmless. Treatment is simple; you should breathe into and out of a paper bag for a few minutes. That will bring the carbon dioxide in your blood back to its correct level and your hand will return to normal.

SEE ALSO

ASTHMA • CRAMPS • NERVOUS SYSTEM • OXYGEN • PAIN

Ice Therapy

Sprains and strains, bruising, and bleeding can all be treated by cooling the injured area with ice. This treatment causes the blood vessels to contract and slows down or stops the bleeding, reduces swelling and inflammation, and helps relieve pain. Applying an ice pack is a quick and efficient way of dealing with many playground and sports injuries.

Making an ice pack is easy. Some crushed ice should be sealed in a plastic bag, which is then placed inside a damp cloth. The cloth should be tied up securely and held gently but firmly over or around the injured area for about 10 minutes. If possible, the injured part of the body should be elevated and rested before and during application of the ice pack. A sterile dressing should be placed over any open wound or scrape before the ice pack is applied. An injured joint should be exercised as soon as the ice pack is removed, to prevent it from becoming too stiff.

Q & A

I cut my lip recently, and it bled a lot for such a tiny wound. Why?

The lips are richly supplied with tiny blood vessels; thus even a small cut can result in much bleeding. Rubbing the cut with an ice cube will constrict the blood vessels, help the blood to clot, and help relieve the pain.

Why does an ankle swell so much if it is sprained?

A minor twist of the ankle when it is bearing the body's weight can result in severe damage to the ligaments that support it. Fluid leaks from the damaged blood vessels into the tissues, and bruising may occur. The swelling can be reduced by using ice to constrict the blood vessels, elevation, and compression with an elasticized bandage.

USES FOR ICE PACKS

Ice packs can be used briefly, and with care, to help bring down a fever. Ice packs are also used in sports clinics and physical therapy departments to relieve pain before and during a session to exercise an injured muscle.

1

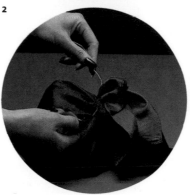

Making an ice pack: (1) Place the ice in a plastic bag and crush it with a mallet or hammer. That allows the pack to contour smoothly to a rounded part of the body. (2) Tie up the bag of crushed ice in a damp cloth, which protects the skin from freeze burn. (3) Apply the pack for about 10 minutes. Any longer than this can burn the skin.

2

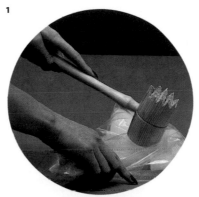

3

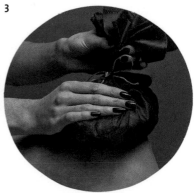

SEE ALSO

BRUISES • CIRCULATORY SYSTEM • SPORTS INJURIES • SPRAINS AND STRAINS

Indigestion

Indigestion is pain or discomfort in the upper abdomen that usually occurs after eating, particularly if the meal includes rich, spicy, or fatty foods. It can occur as a sensation of fullness or nausea, as a gnawing or burning pain, or as a dull ache in the chest, which is sometimes called heartburn. Some people experience an unpleasant acidic taste in the mouth if indigestion continues for some time. The tongue may become dry and coated, and the breath becomes stale.

When the body digests food, the muscles of the stomach squeeze regularly to crush the food. The lining of the stomach produces enzymes and acids, which break the food down further. Then the food passes to the duodenum, where more enzymes digest it before it moves into the intestine. When the stomach is empty, its muscles relax and the lining stops producing the acids and enzymes. The symptoms of indigestion are caused when food remains in the stomach for longer than usual and when substances irritate the lining of the stomach and duodenum. All sorts of items can cause indigestion, among them cucumbers and pickles, creamy dishes, highly spiced foods, caffeine, and alcohol. Eating very quickly, being overweight, and smoking increase the risk of suffering from indigestion. Many people get indigestion when they are stressed or when they take drugs, such as aspirin, that can irritate the digestive tract.

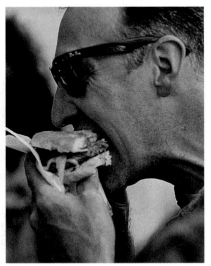

Everyone has indigestion from time to time. If it happens very often, lasts for a long time, or is very severe, it may be a symptom of a more serious stomach disorder, and a doctor should be consulted.

Eating too quickly is one of the easiest ways of getting indigestion. It is best to sit down calmly and chew food slowly to aid digestion. Eating when on the move should be avoided.

Q & A

My father often gets indigestion after he eats a big meal. However, he likes to eat, so what can he do to prevent the indigestion?

The most common causes of indigestion are eating late in the evening, eating spicy or rich foods, eating too much, and drinking alcohol. If your father eats slowly and misses one of the courses, he should be able to reduce his indigestion. If possible, your father should allow at least two hours between eating and his bedtime.

AVOIDANCE AND TREATMENT OF INDIGESTION

Avoid indigestion by
- Eating regularly and slowly
- Chewing food well
- Getting plenty of exercise
- Eating plenty of fiber to avoid constipation
- Avoiding heavy drinking
- Avoiding or reducing spicy foods, greasy foods, and caffeine

Treat indigestion by
- Taking an antacid
- Sipping water and sitting in a cool place, or walking around

SEE ALSO

DIET • DIGESTIVE SYSTEM • DIGESTIVE SYSTEM DISEASES AND DISORDERS • FOOD AND NUTRITION

Iodine

Iodine is a mineral essential for good health, and it is also a necessary component of the hormone thyroxine, which is made in the thyroid gland. Thyroxine is responsible for growth and development and helps maintain the body's vital life-support processes, such as body temperature, use of oxygen, and digestion. If the body produces too much thyroxine, these processes speed up. If too little thyroxine is produced, they slow down. Lack of iodine in adults causes the thyroid gland to enlarge, a condition known as goiter. Myxedema is another disorder caused by lack of iodine. Patients suffering from myxedema become very slow in their actions and gain weight. Their speech and thoughts also slow down. Diseases due to lack of iodine are rare in the Western world.

The body needs only tiny amounts of iodine. Sea salt, fish, and other seafoods are the best sources. Iodine was also once widely used as an antiseptic to clean infected skin.

Q & A

Why do people who live in certain geographical areas seem particularly prone to goiter?

A goiter is a swelling of the thyroid gland. This gland needs a supply of iodine from food or water to produce its hormone, thyroxine. If there is a deficiency of iodine, the thyroid swells. This type of goiter is called endemic goiter. Certain areas of the world, particularly inland mountain regions, lack iodine in the soil and water, so the inhabitants lack iodine, too. In such areas, one must use iodized table salt.

My aunt was given radioactive iodine for an overactive thyroid gland. Was this radiotherapy?

Yes. Unlike other parts of the body, the thyroid gland selectively stores iodine. A drink of radioactive iodine is given to the patient, and the amount of radioactivity that passes into the thyroid gland is sufficient to destroy overactive tissue without harming other parts of the body.

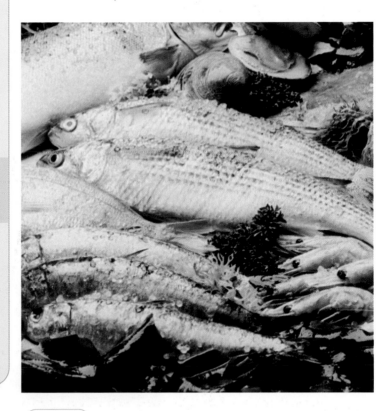

The tiny amounts of iodine that the body needs to function properly are usually provided by foods such as sea fish, shellfish, and sea salt.

SEE ALSO

DIET • GLANDS • GROWTH • MINERALS • NUTRITIONAL DISEASES • SALT • SKIN

Iron

Iron is a mineral that, together with protein, produces hemoglobin. Hemoglobin is a pigmented protein in the red blood cells that transports oxygen from the lungs to the body tissues and gives red blood cells their color. The body does not make iron; it obtains iron from food. The average adult body contains about 0.1–0.14 ounce (3–4 g) of iron. Some of this iron is stored in the liver and spleen; the remainder is present in the red blood cells and in the bone marrow.

Lack of iron in the diet causes anemia, which is one of the most common deficiency disorders in women. An anemic person is constantly tired and unwell. Treatment involves extra iron supplements. Pregnant women need extra iron, as the growing fetus draws on the mother's supply. Although liver, legumes, milk, eggs, wheat germ, and leafy green vegetables are all good sources of iron, large doses of vitamin A have been linked to birth defects, so liver and its products, which contain high levels of this vitamin, should be avoided during pregnancy.

Q & A

Do you lose iron if you give blood regularly?

Yes. If you give blood once every three months, you lose about twice as much iron as normal, but a good mixed diet will replace the loss.

Is it true that spinach contains a lot of iron?

Spinach contains around 0.00012 ounce (4 mg) of iron per 3.5 ounces (100 g) of spinach, which is a moderate amount. Unrefined flour and dried peas and beans contain more iron than most green vegetables, as does meat. The iron in meat is also more easily absorbed by the intestine than the iron in vegetables.

Is it true that iron pills are dangerous for children?

Iron can cause poisoning in infants and children, who should take iron supplements only under strict medical supervision. It is unusual in the United States for children to be given iron pills to treat an iron deficiency. A doctor is more likely to suggest increasing the amount of iron-rich food in the child's diet.

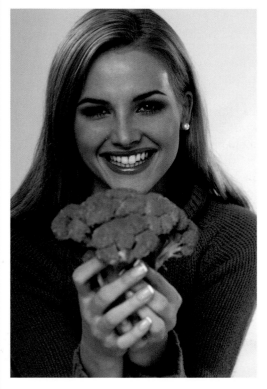

Many young women suffer from iron-deficiency anemia at some time in their life, because of blood loss during menstruation. However, the body can store iron, and if women eat a healthy diet of animal foods and green vegetables, they can avoid anemia. Iron supplements should not be taken unless a doctor prescribes them. Taking too much iron can damage the liver.

SEE ALSO

ANEMIA • MINERALS • NUTRITIONAL DISEASES • VITAMINS

Irritable Bowel Syndrome

Irritable bowel syndrome is a common disorder that features abdominal symptoms for which no organic cause can be found. In the past it was given other various names, such as nervous diarrhea, spastic colon, or idiopathic diarrhea. The term *idiopathic* simply means that the cause is unknown. In the United States, about half the patients seeking medical attention for bowel upset are suffering from irritable bowel syndrome.

Symptoms

The condition usually develops between the ages of 20 and 30 and is twice as common in females as in males, but people of any age and of both sexes can suffer from it. Symptoms are varied and tend to be intermittent. Some pain in the abdomen is usual. Recurrent episodes of pain are commonly localized in one of the four corners of the abdomen and may be relieved by emptying the bowel. The pain may start soon after eating, and many sufferers are convinced that it is brought on by a meal. Eating also often induces an urgent need to use the toilet.

Diarrhea is common and often alternates with constipation, but the condition may involve unduly frequent, but otherwise normal, bowel motions. There may be a constant sense of abdominal fullness and an awareness that something is happening in the intestines. The sufferer is conscious of abdominal noises (borborygmi) and excessive gas production (flatus), and there may be nausea and headache. Sometimes, there is a feeling that there is incomplete emptying of the bowel. Sufferers often notice that the stools are small and rounded or occasionally ribbonlike. Stools may also contain visible mucus. A common feature of the syndrome is anxiety about intestinal function and other health matters.

Normal movement of the bowel contents is brought about by a process known as peristalsis. This is a continuous process organized by a network of nerves in the wall of the intestine, which involves automatic tightening and relaxation of short segments so there is a progressive shifting of the contents in the direction of the rectum. Healthy people are rarely aware of peristalsis, but people suffering from irritable bowel syndrome are acutely conscious of it. This is partly because peristaltic contractions are stronger and more frequent than normal and partly because there is undue awareness of body function.

Causes

People with irritable bowel syndrome are often convinced that they are allergic to certain kinds of food, and that this is the cause of the problem. Food allergy, however, is far less common

Q & A

My sister always has diarrhea and stomach pains before exams. Does she have irritable bowel syndrome, or is this just her nerves acting up because of the exams?

Many people have this kind of reaction before exams. The whole nervous system is affected, and this causes the intestine to become overactive. An irritable intestine causes a similar kind of spasm, but it lasts much longer and may arise without obvious stress.

My doctor thinks I may have irritable bowel syndrome, and he wants me to go to the hospital to have some tests done. I don't like medical tests. Are they really necessary?

There are no symptoms that positively distinguish irritable bowel syndrome from other types of bowel disorders. Diagnosis has to be made by excluding other possible reasons for your symptoms. This can be done only by hospital tests. It does not mean that your doctor is expecting to find anything serious, but having the tests done will provide reassurance.

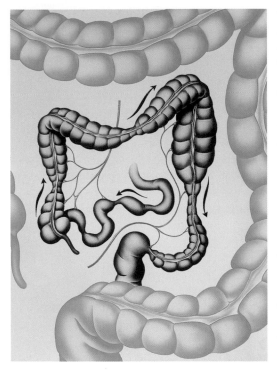

The larger blue structure shows a normal colon; the red one depicts the distension and constriction that is common in irritable bowel syndrome. Muscle movement in the red colon is shown in yellow, and arrows show the direction of the flow of feces.

than is generally supposed, and most doctors do not accept this theory. The syndrome invariably has either a psychological basis or a strong psychological element. It is notoriously common in women of high intelligence and driving ambition, especially those with a tendency to tension and anxiety about professional, financial, and family matters. The syndrome often starts after a life crisis or a period of emotional stress. Many sufferers have developed irritable bowel syndrome after a divorce or a bereavement. In some cases, there is a strong, but not always realized, fear of cancer.

Diagnosis and treatment

Doctors recognize that it can be a serious error to make a premature diagnosis of irritable bowel syndrome without full investigation. Before concluding that a person's symptoms are due entirely to irritable bowel syndrome, it is necessary to exclude a number of other possibilities by carrying out some tests. One of the most important of these is a barium meal X-ray. Barium is an element that X-rays cannot pass through, so it is used to outline internal organs. In irritable bowel syndrome, a barium meal X-ray shows no structural abnormality, but it may indicate an unusual degree of contraction of the circular muscle fibers of the bowel. This suggests that the colon is in a state of abnormally high activity.

Some people with irritable bowel syndrome may require drug treatment to relieve their underlying anxiety. Careful examination to exclude an organic cause, followed by strong reassurance, is often enough to provide a cure. A diet high in vegetable fiber is also helpful in regulating bowel activity. A number of drugs have a specific sedative effect on peristalsis. These calm down excessive contractions in the intestine and relieve abdominal pain.

If patients have psychological symptoms, such as anxiety, the doctor may refer them to a therapist, who can give advice on how to alleviate stress. Some people learn to use mind and body relaxation techniques to help reduce their stress and so improve their bowel symptoms.

SEE ALSO

CONSTIPATION • DIGESTIVE SYSTEM • DIGESTIVE SYSTEM DISEASES AND DISORDERS • PAIN

Isometric Exercises

Q & A

My boyfriend plans to use isometrics to build large biceps. How long should it be before there is an improvement?

If your boyfriend does isometric exercises properly, he should probably be able to feel and measure a change in all the muscles involved after four weeks. However, to achieve the figure of a bodybuilder takes many months of intensive work at isometric exercises, combined with weight lifting and other fitness routines.

I am a football player. Would it help to do some isometric exercises as well as jogging as part of my training?

Yes. Isometrics will help you to develop specific sets of muscles that need to be very strong for your sport.

I would like to become fit. Are isometrics enough?

No. Isometrics are only for building up the muscles. They do not improve the condition of your heart and lungs—one of the main objects of most forms of exercise.

Isometric exercises are a good way to build up muscle over a period of time. They are performed against an immovable object such as a floor, wall, a desktop, or even a fist. Different exercises develop the strength of particular sets of muscles, such as the chest, upper arms, or thighs. The advantage of isometrics is that they can be done anywhere—in the car, at a desk, or wherever a person happens to be. People need to work on the exercises for only about two minutes per day. After about four or five weeks of regular exercise, they will be able to measure the increase in size of the muscles worked on. However, isometric exercises do not help with general physical fitness unless they are combined with other types of exercise that involve the whole body, such as bending, stretching, cycling, and jogging.

Pilates

Pilates is an exercise method developed by Joseph Pilates (1880–1967) to improve physical and mental health. This method focuses on building the body's core strength (back, abdominal, and pelvic muscles) and improving posture through a series of low-repetition, low-impact stretching and conditioning exercises. The aim of Pilates is to provide a complete body workout and develop an awareness of how the body works, enabling the mind and body to work in harmony. Pilates is based on eight principles: relaxation, alignment, control, precision, routine, breathing, centering, and flowing movement.

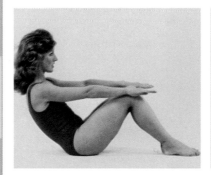 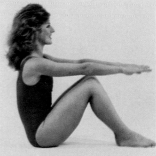

For one type of isometric exercise, lie on the back with the knees bent. Push the feet firmly against the floor, raise the body (left), and bring the arms to knee level and beyond (right). Count to six, relax, and repeat the exercise 10 times.

SEE ALSO

EXERCISE • JOGGING • MUSCLE • PHYSICAL FITNESS • YOGA

Jogging

Q & A

Many of my parents' friends seem to have taken up jogging. Why is it considered such a great fitness activity?

It may seem strange that many people jog as though their life depends on it. Yet a person's life might really depend on jogging, or at least on taking exercise that uses the heart and lungs. Jogging helps to counteract the effects of many things, including stress and a high-fat diet, that contribute to heart disease.

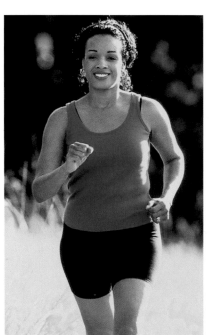

Jogging is a form of exercise that involves running at a slow, steady pace. It is a popular fitness activity for people of all ages that can be done anywhere and at any time. It does not require special training or the use of special sports facilities. All that is needed is a road, track, park, or lane where people can run in safety. Even city dwellers do not usually have a problem fitting jogging into their daily routines. Many men and women, for example, jog to and from work every day or take a daily jog around a local city park. Parents and children often take an early morning jog together.

The benefit of jogging is that it is an aerobic exercise, which helps the body use oxygen more efficiently and strengthens the cardiovascular system (heart, lungs, and circulatory system). Jogging and other aerobic exercises make the heart larger and stronger and, therefore, less prone to disease. Lung capacity is increased, so people are less likely to get out of breath. Metabolism also improves so that waste products, toxins, and excess fat are removed more easily. All this makes people fitter and stronger.

Jogging guidelines

Beginners and overweight people should start jogging gently, building up their fitness gradually. A sensible way to begin is by combining walking with jogging in 15-minute periods. The person then gradually cuts down the walking periods until eventually he or she is jogging for the entire time. It is important to run at a slow, steady pace to exercise the heart and lungs properly. If people jog at a speed at which it is uncomfortable to talk with a friend, they are going too fast. Most adults should have a medical examination before they start to jog. As long as they begin gently, there is very little risk. However, older people who have not exercised for a long time or people with heart problems may be at risk. They should see their doctor before jogging.

Jogging is a popular form of exercise, and if done properly, it can be extremely good for people. The time spent jogging should be built up gradually. Joggers should move at a slow pace, with their whole body, particularly the shoulders, relaxed; comfortable clothes and rubber-soled running shoes should be worn. Joggers should not go too fast—a good test is to be able to talk with a friend as they jog.

SEE ALSO

AEROBICS • BASAL METABOLISM • DIET • EXERCISE • HEART • PHYSICAL FITNESS • SPORTS • SPORTS INJURIES

Joint Disorders

The joints undergo a great deal of wear and tear, so it is not surprising that they suffer from a number of disorders. Some disorders are easily cured with treatment and time, but others may need surgery. Sprains and strains caused by awkward or accidental movements and falls are the most common injuries to joints. They cause swelling and may be extremely painful. These injuries are treated with bandaging and rest of the affected limb.

Knee joint disorders

The knee joint is often injured in sports when it is accidentally twisted and wrenched. It contains two floating pieces of cartilage, which may be torn or crushed. Such an injury causes severe pain and sometimes stops the knee from bending. If this happens too often, the cartilage may have to be removed. In time, the muscles of the knee grow strong enough to take the place of the cartilage.

Sometimes, the whole knee swells after an injury, a condition called water on the knee. Like many other knee problems, it clears up with rest. Too much kneeling on a hard surface or a blow to the knee may cause one of its soft lubricating pads, or bursae, to become inflamed. In this disorder, known as bursitis, or housemaid's knee, a painful, fluid-filled swelling develops in front of the kneecap. Other joints where bursitis may develop include the elbow, the heel, and the base of the big toe.

Dislocations

Accidents may also lead to dislocation, when one bone of a joint is wrenched out of its socket. This displacement prevents normal movement of the joint and is usually extremely painful. The muscles, nerves, and blood vessels around the joint are damaged and the tissues swell. Skilled treatment is needed to reposition the bone as quickly as possible. The shoulder, jaw, and hip are particularly likely to be dislocated.

Spinal joint injuries

The joints of the spine are often injured. The spinal bones (vertebrae) are joined by fibrous tissue. Small disks of pulpy material surrounded by rings of fibrous tissue act as shock absorbers between vertebrae. When the vertebrae are crushed together, as in heavy lifting, the pulp may be forced through the fibrous tissue and press against the spinal cord or a nerve root. This condition is known as a slipped, or prolapsed, disk and can be very painful. Symptoms may come on suddenly or over a period of time. Treatment includes bed rest (lying on a firm mattress for support) and taking painkillers.

Q & A

I dislocated my right shoulder a few months ago. Now it dislocates easily, and I have had to give up playing football. Is there anything I can do to strengthen the joint?

It is possible to have an operation, known as the Putti-Platt operation, to increase the strength of the joint if a shoulder repeatedly dislocates. This procedure builds up the bone at the front of the shoulder to increase the depth of the socket, making it more difficult for the bone to slip out. Healing takes about two months.

I am double-jointed. Am I more likely to develop rheumatism when I get older?

People who are said to be double-jointed do not, in fact, have double joints. They do have greater than normal flexibility and can move their bodies and limbs through a wider range of movement than most people. As a result, their joints are subjected to unusual stresses and strains through overuse. "Double-jointed" people may be more prone to aches and pains in their joints later in life.

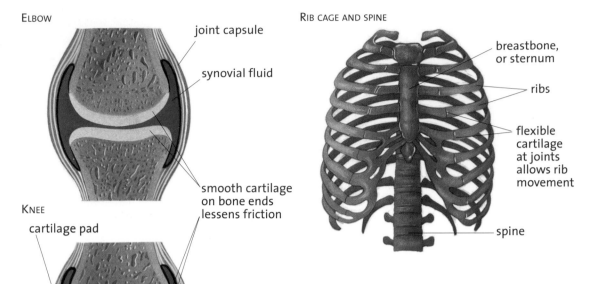

ELBOW

joint capsule

synovial fluid

smooth cartilage
on bone ends
lessens friction

KNEE

cartilage pad

RIB CAGE AND SPINE

breastbone,
or sternum

ribs

flexible
cartilage
at joints
allows rib
movement

spine

*Highly mobile joints, which include the
elbow (top left) and the knee (bottom
left) are particularly susceptible to injury.
These joints are enclosed within fibrous
tissue, known as the joint capsule, and
contain synovial fluid, which acts as a
lubricant. The knee joint also contains
shock-absorbing cartilage pads. Certain
joints on each of the ribs (top right),
however, are formed from bone and
cartilage. These cartilaginous joints allow
movement without the need for fluid-
filled synovial membranes, as in the
elbow and knee.*

Other joint disorders

Inflammation of the synovial membrane that lines a joint can be
caused by an injury or by rheumatoid arthritis. Sometimes, it can
lead to ankylosis, or permanent fixation of the joint. This most
often affects the area around the spine and the pelvis. The joints
may also be affected by osteoarthritis, which causes the cartilage
around them to wear away gradually.

People whose joints are badly worn away, creating pain and
limiting movement, can now be fitted with new joints made of
metal, plastic, or ceramic. These artificial joints help relieve the
pain, and, with exercise and practice, the patient may, in time,
regain full movement of the joint.

Rheumatism

Rheumatism is a term used to describe a range of aches and
pains. It is not a disease in itself; it is more a collection of
symptoms. The aches and pains, including swelling, tenderness,
and stiffness, affect the joints and other surrounding structures,
such as muscles, tendons, and ligaments.

SEE ALSO

ARTHRITIS • ELBOW • FRACTURES AND DISLOCATIONS • HIP
• JOINT REPLACEMENT • JOINTS • KNEE • LEG • LIGAMENTS •
MUSCLE • MUSCLE DISEASES AND DISORDERS • SHOULDER •
SKELETAL SYSTEM • SPORTS INJURIES • SPRAINS AND STRAINS
• TENDON

Joint Replacement

Q & A

When a joint is replaced, is the new joint from a human donor?

No. Replacement joints are always artificial.

Which joints can be replaced?

Most replacement operations involve the hip and the knee. However, joints have been designed for the finger and toe joints; the elbow, shoulder, and ankle; and the articulation of the jaw (the temporomandibular joint in front of each ear).

Do artificial joints last for a lifetime?

That depends on the recipient's age. Many new joints perform well for the rest of a person's life, but loosening of the attachment to the bones and other problems sometimes occur. Such problems may require a further operation.

What does a joint revision operation involve?

Joint revision involves opening up the joint site, removing any loose or damaged artificial parts, and replacing them with new parts.

Joint replacement refers to a type of operation in which a diseased or damaged joint, such as a knee, is removed and replaced by an artificial, or prosthetic, joint. In the past, people often became less mobile as they aged, because accumulated damage to the joints caused so much pain that they could not bear to move. However, joint replacement has given many people the ability to enjoy an active life well into their senior years.

Joints are structures where two or more bones, bone and cartilage, or bone and teeth come together. They are usually held together by a series of muscles, ligaments, and tendons. Some joints allow no movement; others allow movement to a greater or lesser degree. Joints that allow a significant amount of movement often include layers of cartilage between the bones to prevent them from grinding against each other. They are also often enclosed within sacs filled with fluid to lubricate and cushion the joint to ease movement.

Joints that allow movement are the ones subject to the greatest wear and tear over the course of life. Not surprisingly, they are the ones that are most often replaced. Hip, knee, and ankle joints top the list of those that are replaced, because of their importance in walking and in supporting the weight of the body. Other joints that are frequently rebuilt include the shoulder and the many joints in the hand and wrist.

Damage to the joints can result from overuse, injuries, failure to heal properly after an injury has occurred, or from chronic or infectious diseases. Arthritis, old age, obesity, and repetitive stress all contribute to the need for joint replacement.

The procedure

Joint replacement is often a last resort; medication and physical therapy are less drastic and less risky treatments for joint pain. However, when joint damage is so severe that pain cannot be managed or when it is so severe that it limits the daily activities of the individual, surgery becomes a more desirable option.

During surgery, the damaged or diseased bone and cartilage are removed. The affected area is cleaned out and prepared for insertion and attachment of the prosthesis (replacement joint), which is made of metal, plastics, ceramics, or some kind of composite material. The muscles and tendons are then attached to the prosthesis, and the site is closed.

After surgery, the joint is immobilized for some time to avoid damage to the prosthesis as well as the remaining tissue. Inflammation, a natural response to injury, must be controlled to prevent swelling of the tissues, which restricts the blood supply vital to the healing process. Pain also has to be managed.

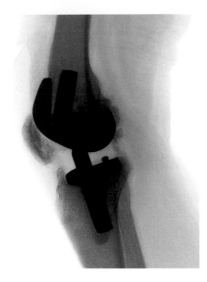

This X-ray of the knee shows a side view of an artificial replacement. The component parts of the new joint are fixed into the femur, or thighbone, and the tibia, or shinbone.

Taken after a hip replacement operation, this X-ray shows a metal component screwed into the femur (thighbone) to strengthen it. (The zipper and buckle of the patient's trousers appear at the left.)

Once the patient is well enough, physical therapy and training are very important, because the person must learn how to live and move with an artificial joint. Appropriate exercise increases the strength of surrounding muscles and promotes healing by increasing blood flow to the site of the operation.

Potential complications

Joint replacement surgery is not without risk. Patients who have their hips, knees, or ankles replaced are at increased risk of blood clots. That can lead to potentially fatal complications, such as pulmonary embolisms (in which the blood clot comes loose and is transported to the lungs). Infections are always a potential complication of surgery, as is excess bleeding or pneumonia. Prostheses may become displaced from their proper position or may break free entirely. Abnormal bone growth adjacent to the prosthesis may also be a problem.

Joint replacements are rarely a onetime event. Over time, revision surgery is typically necessary to repair or replace worn parts of the prosthesis. Depending on the type of prosthesis and the level of a person's activity, the time before subsequent surgery is required may be 10 to 20 years. Ongoing improvements in methods and materials may eventually extend this period.

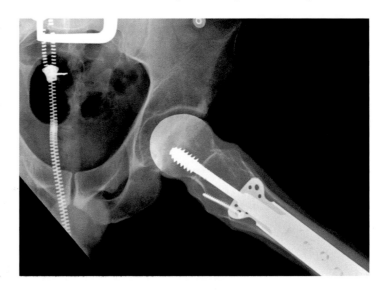

SEE ALSO

AGING • ARTHRITIS • CALCIUM • ELBOW • FRACTURES AND DISLOCATIONS • HIP • JOINT DISORDERS • JOINTS • KNEE • LEG • ORTHOPEDICS • PAIN • SHOULDER • SKELETAL SYSTEM

Joints

The body contains more than 200 bones, which are linked by joints. Some joints are fixed: the bones of the skull, for instance, are bound together by fibrous tissue and cannot move. Other joints are lined with a tough elastic tissue called cartilage and allow great movement and flexibility. To avoid friction, movable joints are lubricated, or kept moist, by fluid from the synovial membrane, which surrounds the joints.

There are various kinds of movable joints. The joints of the fingers, elbows, and knees are known as hinge joints. They can move backward and forward. Pivot joints, such as those at the top of the neck, allow rotary movements, such as turning the head. Gliding joints, such as those of the spine, wrists, and feet, allow a sliding movement. Ball-and-socket joints, such as those of the hip and shoulder, enable the bones to move in all directions.

The knee joint is one of the more complicated joint structures (more than it would first appear), and it is one of the joints most commonly injured by athletes.

The knee joint

When a person extends his or her knee beyond the straight position, it locks. This locking is brought about by a very slight but important twisting movement of the large bone (the tibia) in the lower part of the leg. There are two pieces of cartilage, called semilunar cartilages, that pad between the cartilage linings of the femur (thighbone). One piece of cartilage wedges the outside of the joint, and the other wedges the inside of the joint.

The outer edge of each semilunar cartilage is attached to two extremely strong ligaments, one running down the outside of the leg and one running down the inside. These ligaments form the lateral and medial colateral ligaments of the knee, with the cartilage forming a sandwich between them. Any twisting movement of the knee that pulls the ligaments can tear the cartilage. A torn cartilage causes severe pain and sometimes an inability to bend the knee.

The knee also has two ligaments, called the anterior and posterior cruciate ligaments, in the center of the joint for added stability. One ligament crosses from front to back and the other crosses from back to front. These ligaments are also vulnerable to tearing, particularly if the knee is dislocated.

SEE ALSO

ELBOW • HIP • JOINT DISORDERS • JOINT REPLACEMENT • KNEE • SHOULDER • SKELETAL SYSTEM • SLIPPED DISK • SPORTS INJURIES • SPRAINS AND STRAINS

Q & A

Is it true that muscles can restrict a joint's movement against the person's will?

Yes. Limitation of joint movement usually results when the surrounding muscles go into spasm because of pain. This is a protective mechanism to stop the joint from becoming dislocated and to minimize the effects of any injury.

My brother can crack his finger joints like gunfire, driving me completely crazy. Besides being annoying, isn't this bad for his fingers?

No damage occurs from cracking the finger joints. The noise is caused by a slipping of the lateral tendons that hold the joints in place around the bone ends. The tendons slip back into position after a little time.

Are there really some joints that don't move at all?

Yes. The bony plates that make up the skull are fastened tightly together by fixed joints called sutures. These joints are movable in a newborn baby but quickly knit together.

Junk Food

Junk food is food that contains many nutritionally undesirable ingredients, such as saturated fats and refined sugar, and relatively little fiber or vitamins. Junk food is often easily available or quick to prepare. Fast food, bought for takeout meals, is often called junk food. It includes burgers, french fries, hot dogs, pizzas, fried chicken, and carbonated drinks.

Preserving agents, as well as artificial flavoring and coloring, are also added to some junk foods. A 10-ounce (300-ml) milk shake, for example, is often made with only 5 ounces (150 ml) of milk, topped with air, texturizer, coloring, and artificial flavoring. A half-pound (200-g) hamburger contains almost two-thirds of the body's daily fat needs. A large can of soda may have as much as 12 teaspoons of added sugar.

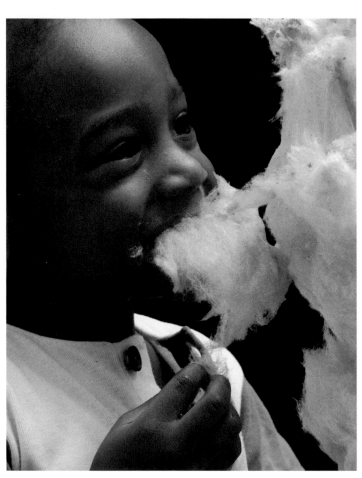

Nutritionists say that people who rely on a regular diet of junk food are endangering their health. Too many calories in the form of fat can increase weight and can lead to heart problems and some forms of cancer. The refined sugar in soft drinks is also high in calories. Too many of these drinks can result in tooth decay, weight gain, and a number of diseases. Food and drink additives can cause headaches and dizziness. Many food additives seem to be linked with hyperactivity in young children, although this link has not been proved.

Most young people enjoy junk food, and a little does no harm. However, if eaten regularly in place of healthy, fresh food, it is detrimental to health. If someone eats a balanced diet most of the time, the occasional junk food meal will have no lasting ill effects.

This little girl is eating cotton candy. Cotton candy tastes good but contains no vitamins—just the empty calories of sugar. Eating too much junk food can take away the appetite for healthier food.

SEE ALSO

CALORIES • CARBOHYDRATES • DIET • FATS • FOOD ADDITIVES • FOOD AND NUTRITION • HEALTH FOODS • NUTRITIONAL DISEASES • OBESITY • SUGARS • WEIGHT CONTROL

Knee

The knee is the largest joint in the human body. It is strong enough to hold the body upright and enables the lower leg to move, allowing humans to walk and run.

The knee lies between the thighbone (femur) and shin bone (tibia). It is designed like a hinge to allow forward and backward movement. The rounded end of the femur rests in the saucer-shaped top of the tibia. A smooth substance called cartilage coats the ends of both these bones to help prevent friction. Further protection against damage is provided by pads of cartilage on either side of the knee joint. A small triangular bone, called the kneecap or patella, lies embedded in the tendon in front of the knee.

Special fluid, called synovial fluid, is contained in a capsule surrounding the whole joint. This lubricates (moistens) the bones to prevent friction. Strong ligaments hold the knee joint in place. The thigh muscles control the knee's movement; those at the front straighten the knee, and those at the rear pull it back.

The knee is highly susceptible to injuries, especially in people who take part in sports. Knee injuries include strains, torn cartilage, and a dislocated kneecap.

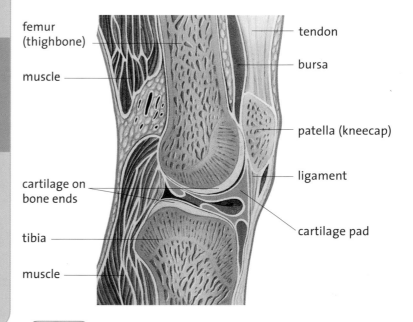

femur (thighbone) — muscle — cartilage on bone ends — tibia — muscle — tendon — bursa — patella (kneecap) — ligament — cartilage pad

This side view of the knee shows the internal structure of the joint in detail, including the soft tissues.

SEE ALSO

FRACTURES AND DISLOCATIONS • JOINT DISORDERS • JOINT REPLACEMENT • JOINTS • LIGAMENTS • MUSCLE • SKELETAL SYSTEM • SPORTS INJURIES • SPRAINS AND STRAINS

Leg

Q & A

My brother has been told that he will not be able to play soccer for a while because of damage to his Achilles tendon. What is this?

The Achilles tendon is attached to the heel and is the link between the foot and the powerful calf muscles at the back of the leg. These muscles provide the power for walking and running; when they contract, they pull on the tendon and the heel is raised. This tendon is extremely strong, but occasionally it gets torn. Surgery is the only means of repair, and a fairly long convalescence is usually needed.

A car accident has left me with one leg shorter than the other. Can the short leg be corrected by a bone graft?

It might be possible. In a bone graft, pieces of bone are taken from elsewhere in the person's body, or from a donor. The grafted bone is used as a supporting structure around which new bone can develop. Usually it is not possible to make up more than 2 inches (5 cm) in length by bone grafting; a longer section of grafted bone would be too weak.

The legs enable people to stand, walk, run, and jump. The femur, or thighbone, is the largest and strongest bone in the body. At its top end, the femur fits comfortably into the hip bone to form a ball-and-socket joint that allows the leg to move in all directions. At its lower end, the femur meets the lower leg bones to form the knee joint. This is a hinge joint that allows the lower leg to swing back and forth. There are two long bones in the lower leg. These are the tibia, or shinbone, which is the heavier of the two, and the narrower fibula. The tibia and the fibula are joined together by ligaments. At the foot, these two bones are joined to the ankle, which is a flexible joint like the wrist.

Soft tissue

The soft tissue of the leg consists of muscle interlaced with nerves and blood vessels. Thigh muscles work in groups with those of the hip to allow the legs to bend and straighten during movement. The thigh muscles also give stability, holding the body balanced upright when a person is standing. Muscles in the calf, attached to the knee and ankle joints by strong tendons, also help steady the legs when people stand. These lower leg muscles also control movement of the feet.

The sciatic nerve that runs down the outside of each leg is the largest nerve in the body. It supplies nerve impulses from the spinal cord to the hip, some thigh muscles, and the muscles of the lower leg.

Blood supply

Blood is supplied to the legs by the femoral artery and returns to the heart through two sets of veins, one set deep inside the leg, the other nearer the surface. The walls of the veins in the leg are thinner than artery walls. Blood has to travel upward toward the heart, so the journey puts considerable pressure on the veins. They are equipped with one-way valves to prevent the blood from flowing backward.

Leg disorders

Among the most common leg disorders is arthritis of the knee or hip, which usually occurs because of wear and tear on the joint. Broken leg bones and damage to the soft tissues of the knee and hip are common in people who take part in vigorous sports.

With age the valves in the leg veins can become damaged, leading to varicose veins. In this condition, the blood flows backward in the veins, causing swelling and tenderness. Other leg problems include ankle injuries, sciatica (inflammation of the sciatic nerve), and artery disorders.

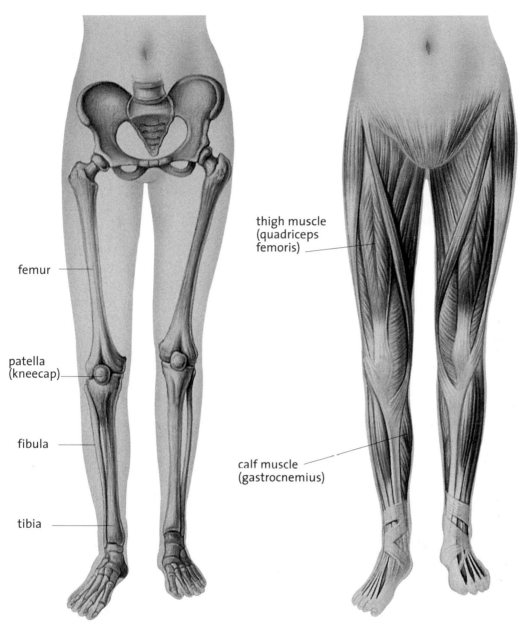

femur

patella
(kneecap)

fibula

tibia

thigh muscle
(quadriceps
femoris)

calf muscle
(gastrocnemius)

The leg bones are the longest and heaviest in the body. The muscles of the leg are also powerful. Those of the thigh act with the hip to give stability and balance. The calf muscles are used in walking, to steady the legs when standing, and to control foot movement.

SEE ALSO

ARTHRITIS • CIRCULATORY SYSTEM • CRAMPS • FEET • FRACTURES AND DISLOCATIONS • HIP • JOINTS • KNEE • LIGAMENTS • MUSCLE • MUSCLE DISEASES AND DISORDERS • SCIATICA • SKELETAL SYSTEM

Lethargy

The term *lethargy*, implying a state of drowsiness, is derived from the Greek word *lethargos*, meaning "forgetful." The term is now generally used to mean indifference to events, a general lack of inclination to undertake any activity, or an abnormal lack of energy. In the opinion of many parents, lethargy is a frequent feature of teenage life, and it is true that young people can sometimes appear to be dull, apathetic, listless, and sluggish.

Social causes of lethargy

In a few cases, lethargy is a symptom of an organic or psychological disorder, but the great majority of cases are the result of social factors over which young people may feel they have little or no control. However, this is not necessarily the case.

Lethargy and apathy are often seen as separate conditions. However, although these words are usually defined to suggest that lethargy is a physical state and apathy is a mental state, the conditions are often inseparable. The relationship between the mind and the body is so interwoven that it is virtually impossible for something to happen to one without affecting the other. One of the main causes of lethargy, when it occurs as an abnormal lack of energy or motivation, is apathy—an absence of interest or enthusiasm. A lively relish for life is one of the most valuable qualities humans can have, and, for many young people, severe lethargy may be due to lack of interest or participation in events or ideas.

Interest, motivation, and creativity are also closely linked. A person who has become intensely interested in a topic, whatever it may be, will want to become engaged in it and will want to do something with it. Not everyone has the talent or inclination to paint pictures, compose music, create computer programs, or write the great American novel. However, those who have developed an interest in such activities find that, once the creative impulse is fully aroused, lethargy disappears.

The physical passivity of lethargy also affects the mind adversely, because everything that happens to the body affects the mind. Those who are inactive are likely to develop an inactive mind. Research has shown that most people who engage in strenuous physical activity, such as sports or athletics, have high morale and an optimistic mental outlook.

Medical causes of lethargy

Lethargy and apathy are characteristic of many serious diseases, especially kidney failure, blood poisoning (septicemia), brain abscess, AIDS, typhoid fever, typhus, hypothermia, exhaustion, and heavy worm infestation. However, some medical causes of

Q & A

I've put on weight and feel drowsy all the time and completely lacking in energy. Could this be caused by a problem with my glands?

It is unlikely. In rare cases, however, lethargy can be a symptom of endocrine system disorders such as myxedema (a failure of the thyroid gland to produce enough thyroid hormone). In such cases, lethargy is accompanied by weight gain, and the menstrual cycle is often disturbed. When lethargy is due to a disturbance of the hormone glands, there are usually other symptoms that point to this as a cause. Check with your doctor.

I've heard that I should expect to grow more lethargic as I grow older. Is that true?

No. You may find that your physical capacities grow more limited as a result of the aging process, but you should not suffer from lethargy. Maintaining energy is a question of having plenty to do and keeping your body in good shape by exercising. You should also keep your brain alert, as lethargy can be the result of boredom.

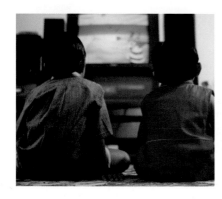

Watching television should not be the main leisure occupation for children. A measured amount of viewing mixed with plenty of stimulating activities is a good way to ward off lethargy.

lethargy are less apparent and can affect young people. For example, clinical depression is an important cause of lethargy. It should be distinguished from the normal depressed mental state that accompanies physical lethargy from social causes. Clinical (pathological) depression is a serious and dangerous state featuring sadness out of proportion to any external cause, self-reproach, loss of self-esteem, and, often, suicidal tendencies. It requires urgent medical attention. The same applies to schizophrenia, a mental illness that usually starts in the teenage years. If lethargy or apathy is associated with evidence of delusions (irrational beliefs or ideas) and hallucinations, which occur when a person experiences a sensation that has no physical cause, such as hearing voices or seeing nonexistent entities, schizophrenia may be suspected.

Sometimes, lethargy is caused by an underactive thyroid gland. The thyroid gland produces hormones that act on almost every cell in the body, prompting it to activity. A severe lack of thyroid hormone produces marked slowing of mind and body; severe lethargy and apathy; dry, scaly, thickened, and coarse skin; cessation of menstruation in women; and a drop in body temperature. Treatment with replacement thyroid hormone reverses these symptoms.

Other causes of lethargy

Psychological conditions associated with lethargy are post-traumatic stress syndrome, chronic fatigue syndrome, alcohol- or drug related social problems, anorexia nervosa, and bulimia. Persistent, heavy use of marijuana (cannabis) can induce a condition known as the motivational syndrome, a state of apathy in which there is an unwillingness to do anything and a tendency to drop out of educational and other activities. Lethargy often accompanies loss of ambition and interest.

Many women find that the changes in the hormonal balance each month can induce mood changes that lead to lethargy. Lethargy is also common in the early weeks of pregnancy and again in the first weeks of a baby's life, when the mother is having to cope with hormonal changes and the stress of caring for a newborn baby. Infectious diseases, viral illnesses, and lack of sleep also lead to feelings of lethargy.

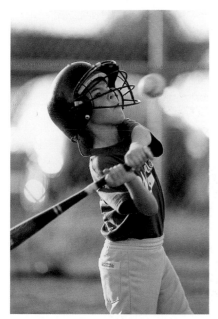

Playing a game such as baseball is a healthy way to enjoy fresh air and get exercise, and it is an invigorating alternative to doing nothing at all.

SEE ALSO

AGING • ANOREXIA AND BULIMIA • EXERCISE • GLANDS • SKIN • SPORTS • TIREDNESS

Ligaments

Ligaments are strong, straplike bands of connective tissue. They bind bones together at the joints and, like the hinges of a door, prevent the joints from moving too far. Without ligaments, bones would be dislocated very easily. Sheets of ligaments hold internal organs such as the kidneys and spleen in place, and fine strands of ligaments give support to the breasts. Ligaments are both tough and yielding. They consist of bundles of fiber made up of a tough, white protein called collagen and smaller amounts of a more elastic protein called elastin. Ligaments suffer damage if they are stretched too far. Injuries include sprains and strains, particularly of the knee, wrist, ankle, and shoulder. Ligaments may also tear or become detached from the bone. Treatment includes rest, ice therapy, and supportive bandages. Most injuries heal easily. In severe cases, surgery may be necessary.

Q & A

My father enjoys squash, but he keeps dislocating his shoulder whenever he tries to play. Can his ligaments be strengthened?

Ligaments are not elastic, so it is a question of their being shortened, not strengthened. Recurrent dislocation can also be due to muscular deficiencies or problems in the joint, so your father should see his doctor for a checkup. Stretched ligaments can shorten, but they need rest; playing squash may be aggravating the problem. If necessary, some ligaments can be shortened surgically.

My sister has terrible posture. Could this be because her ligaments are slack?

Many ligaments become stretched as a result of long-term poor posture, but this is an effect, not a cause. Unless there is a structural abnormality, poor posture is usually due to poor habits. When people allow their postural muscles to weaken, the ligaments have to bear the strain and this gradually stretches them. Postural reeducation and exercise will help your sister to improve her posture.

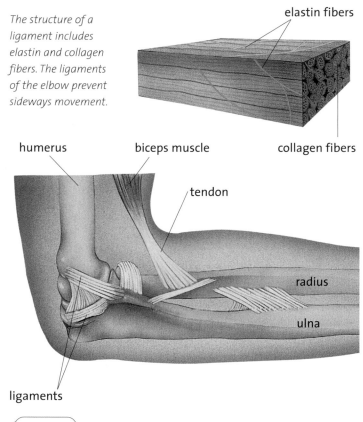

The structure of a ligament includes elastin and collagen fibers. The ligaments of the elbow prevent sideways movement.

elastin fibers

collagen fibers

humerus

biceps muscle

tendon

radius

ulna

ligaments

SEE ALSO

ELBOW • HIP • ICE THERAPY • JOINT DISORDERS • JOINTS • KNEE • LEG • MUSCLE • SHOULDER • SPORTS INJURIES • SPRAINS AND STRAINS • TENDON

Malnutrition

Malnutrition is any form of poor health caused by not eating enough food or by eating the wrong kind of food in the wrong amount. People should eat appropriate quantities of quality food, and it should contain all the vitamins, proteins, carbohydrates, fats, and minerals needed to keep the body healthy. In developed countries, obesity due to a poor diet with high levels of fat and lots of junk food is a type of malnutrition. Elderly people and hospital patients may also suffer from malnutrition, because they may not be able to look after themselves properly and may be too weak or ill to eat properly.

The most obvious malnutrition, however, is the starvation that occurs in some countries in the developing world. Their food generally lacks protein, and there may be far less food than people need. In many countries, half the children die before they reach the age of five. Conditions are made worse by famine, drought, and war. These countries cannot afford to import food. Moreover, it often proves difficult to distribute donated food to those who most need it. As a result, people suffer from varying degrees of starvation and do not get enough nutritious food to maintain health.

Lack of protein

The most common cause of malnutrition is lack of protein, which occurs in some African countries. Kwashiorkor and marasmus are two diseases that afflict young children. Weight loss; retarded growth; wasted muscles; dry, inelastic, cold skin; and sparse hair are typical symptoms of these diseases. Antibodies are made of proteins, and a severe shortage of protein therefore results in a failure to make antibodies. That causes severe immune deficiency and probable death from infection. If treated early with a diet based on milk and high-calorie food supplements, protein-deficiency diseases can be cured.

Voluntary starvation

Few people endure starvation out of choice. Some, however, fast for dietary or religious reasons, and such fasting can cause severe malnutrition if practiced regularly. Anorexia nervosa is a starvation disease that is common in young girls who begin dieting to lose weight. Soon, losing weight becomes a compulsion, and the sufferer may take appetite suppressants and laxatives. If untreated, anorexia nervosa can result in death.

The elderly

As people grow older they generally become more frail and experience loss of strength and balance. It is therefore

When a child suffers from malnutrition, the limbs may become wasted while the belly is distended. The child becomes more and more lethargic, and the face becomes pinched and gray, with sunken eyes. This condition is known as marasmus. The most common cause is starvation, although marasmus can also be a symptom of certain illnesses that stop the child from taking in nourishment from his or her food.

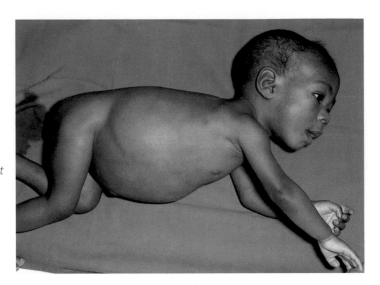

particularly important that the elderly eat sufficient amounts of suitable food, including protein, selected vitamins, and dietary supplements to help overcome these effects of aging.

Studies have shown that a lack of specific nutrients—including protein; vitamins A, D, and C; and the B vitamin folate—increases the risk of becoming frail. As people age, their ability to absorb nutrients from food also decreases. In addition, many elderly people may have a fixed income, which affects the quality and quantity of the food eaten. However, frailty may be easily prevented and even reversed: meat, beans, and nuts are excellent sources of protein and folate, and fruits and vegetables are good sources of vitamins A, C, and D.

Treatment

Malnutrition is treated, whenever possible, by gradually giving the patient a full, balanced diet (a sudden change in eating patterns could be too much for a malnourished body to cope with). Sometimes, vitamin and mineral supplements may be necessary for a while, and any medical problems need to be treated. Normally, however, there is no need to take extra vitamins or minerals, and they can even be harmful. Eating properly should provide all the nourishment needed.

> **SEE ALSO**
>
> ANOREXIA AND BULIMIA • DIET • FOOD AND NUTRITION •
> JUNK FOOD • MILK • MINERALS • NUTRITIONAL DISEASES •
> OBESITY • PROTEIN • VITAMINS

Massage

Massage is a treatment often used for dancers, athletes such as football players, and anyone else who engages in strenuous activity. It is used to help relieve the stiffness that is associated with hard exercise and stops the muscles from becoming too taut. Massage also promotes relaxation and reduces tension and stress in the body.

There are different types of massage designed to soothe and stimulate the body's tissues, muscles, and ligaments. Professional masseurs and masseuses are trained in the techniques to use on different parts of the body and for different conditions.

Massage works by stimulating the circulation of the blood and the functioning of the nervous system. During exercise, waste products are released into the muscles. They often cause stiffness after exercise. It can take several days before waste products are eliminated from the body. Massage speeds up this process by stimulating the lymphatic system and blood circulation. The soothing movements also appear to help lower blood pressure.

A massage can relieve headaches and release muscle tension, promoting relaxation and calm. Many people with stressful jobs have a regular massage, because it promotes mental and physical well-being in a natural, drug-free way.

Q & A

Is a massage carried out for cosmetic purposes the same as a massage used in medicine?

If massage is used to help someone lose weight, it may be very similar to massage for medical purposes. However, facial massage, which is helpful for wrinkles, skin tone, and tension, is very light. The facial muscles are thin, and the rich supply of blood and lymph vessels to this area will respond better to light stroking motions than to pressure, which would be painful.

Are mechanical massagers good?

Electrical vibration massagers can be helpful, especially for self-massage. The vibration can accomplish many of the same effects as manual massage and is useful for breaking up deposits of fat and improving the blood circulation. The best such massagers, although expensive, are the ones that strap onto the back of the hand, allowing the sensitivity and contact of the hands to direct the movement. However, an electrical massager should never be used on bony areas.

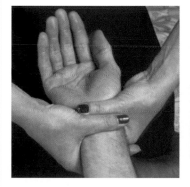 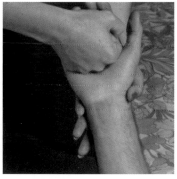

Almost any part of the body can be massaged to induce a feeling of well-being. A number of different movements are used in massage. They include gentle pressure, kneading with the knuckles and the palms of the hands, rolling muscles between the hands, applying friction with the thumbs, and gentle twisting and pulling movements.

SEE ALSO

BLOOD PRESSURE • CIRCULATORY SYSTEM • EXERCISE • LIGAMENTS • MUSCLE • NERVOUS SYSTEM • PHYSICAL FITNESS • PHYSICAL THERAPY • REST AND RELAXATION

Milk

Milk is an extremely valuable food. It contains carbohydrates, fats, and protein. It is also rich in vitamin A, vitamin D, calcium, and phosphorus. An 8-ounce (227-g) glass of milk provides about one-third of the daily requirement of calcium. Calcium helps build and maintain strong bones and teeth. This mineral also plays an important role in nerve function, muscle contraction, and blood clotting. The protein in milk contains all of the essential amino acids in the proportions that the body requires for good health.

Most children and adults drink cow's milk, although goat's milk and buffalo milk are drunk in some parts of the world. A baby drinks human milk from its mother's breasts; human milk provides all the nourishment the baby needs in the first few weeks or months of life. Breast milk contains antibodies that help protect the baby from infections. Milk preparations for bottle-fed babies contain the same nutrients but no antibodies.

Although cow's milk is an important source of protein and calcium, it is not a complete food for growing children and adults. They need to add other proteins, vitamins, fiber, and carbohydrates to their diets. Whole milk also contains a lot of fat (cream), which is not good for health. Nutritionists now believe that it is better to drink low-fat or skim milk, from which most of the cream has been removed.

Q & A

Why does my doctor suggest I drink low-fat milk?

Dairy products, including milk, can be high in saturated fat, which can raise blood cholesterol levels and increase your risk of heart disease. By drinking low-fat milk, you will reduce your risk of these health problems.

My grandmother insists that I should drink a lot of milk. Why? What are the benefits?

Milk contains a large amount of calcium, a mineral that your body needs to build strong bones and teeth. During adolescence, bones grow rapidly, so a teenager in particular needs to make sure that his or her diet includes enough calcium to guarantee the growth of strong bones. A teenager needs about 0.05 ounce (1.3 g) of calcium per day. If a person does not get enough calcium in his or her diet, the body will take calcium from the bones for use in other parts of the body.

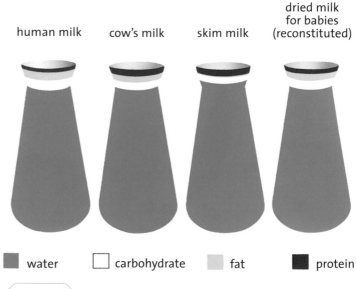

human milk   cow's milk   skim milk   dried milk for babies (reconstituted)

■ water   ☐ carbohydrate   ■ fat   ■ protein

Milk preparations for babies have amounts of fat, carbohydrate, and protein similar to those in human milk. Cow's milk, whether whole or skim, does not.

SEE ALSO

CALCIUM • CARBOHYDRATES • DIET • FATS • FOOD AND NUTRITION • GROWTH • MINERALS • NUTRITIONAL DISEASES • PROTEIN • SUGARS • VITAMINS

Minerals

Minerals such as iron, copper, and zinc are present in the body in minute quantities and are vital for health. These minerals (and many others) are present in the soil, where they are extracted by plants. Humans obtain the minerals from fruits and vegetables or from meat and dairy products (derived from animals that feed on plants). Minerals are essential for maintaining mental and physical health. In the human body, minerals perform a wide range of functions, but a healthy, balanced diet will probably provide all the necessary minerals. A lack of iron is one of the most common mineral deficiencies, particularly in developing countries. Older people sometimes develop a zinc deficiency. Extra minerals should not be taken except when prescribed by a doctor. All minerals can be poisonous if they are taken in excess; iron tablets, for example, can cause serious poisoning in young children.

MINERALS AND THEIR USES IN THE BODY

MINERAL	ROLE	SOURCE
Calcium	Essential in the structure and working of bones and muscles; important in nerve functioning	Dairy produce, eggs, vegetables
Chromium	Essential for the handling of sugar	Fats, meat, vegetable oils
Copper	Needed for the absorption of iron	Seafood, liver, nuts, cereals
Fluoride (fluorine)	Helps protect the teeth against decay	Water
Iodine	Required for thyroid activity	Seafood, vegetables; commonly added to table salt
Iron	Required to make hemoglobin and prevent anemia	Meat, egg yolks, green vegetables, cereals
Magnesium	Important for many body processes; enables the cells to use oxygen	Green vegetables, nuts, cereals
Manganese	Needed for the control of fats in the body and for the cells to use oxygen	Green vegetables, cereals
Phosphorus (phosphate)	Basic energy store in body cells; also works with calcium in bones and muscles	Meat, dairy products, fish, legumes, cereals
Potassium	Acts with sodium to control all electrical activity in the body; required by all tissues	Fresh fruits and vegetables
Sodium chloride (common salt)	Essential component of all organisms; present in all tissues; maintains balance of body fluids	All foods; added during cooking
Zinc	Required for many organisms; present in all tissues; maintains balance of body fluids	Seafood, meat, nuts

SEE ALSO

ANEMIA • DIET • FOOD AND NUTRITION • IRON • SALT

Motor Neuron Disease

Q & A

What exactly is a motor neuron?

A neuron is a nerve cell. It has a small, spiky body and a long nerve fiber called an axon. Sensory neurons carry nerve information to the brain, and motor neurons carry activating signals from the brain to the muscles and glands.

Are the sensory nerves affected in motor neuron disease?

No; only the motor nerves are affected. There is no reduction in sensation, and there is no disturbance of mental functioning.

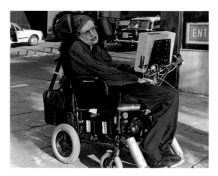

The distinguished British physicist Stephen Hawking (b. 1942) has suffered from amyotrophic lateral sclerosis for nearly 40 years. He still writes books and gives lectures with the help of a speech synthesizer and computer.

Motor neuron disease (amyotrophic lateral sclerosis) is often called Lou Gehrig's disease after the U.S. baseball player Lou Gehrig (1903–1941), who died from it. The cause of this form of motor neuron disease is usually unknown, but in a small minority of people there is a genetic cause. The term *motor neuron disease*, however, covers several similar conditions, of which amyotrophic lateral sclerosis is the most serious.

There are two groups of motor neurons or nerves: the upper motor neurons and the lower motor neurons. The upper motor neurons run downward from the surface of the brain, through the brain and the brain stem and down the spinal cord to end in a series of junctions positioned at the front of the cord from top to bottom. The lower motor neurons emerge from these junctions to run to and activate the muscles. Motor neuron disease may affect either the upper or the lower neurons, or both.

Amyotrophic lateral sclerosis is a combined upper and lower motor neuron disease. It is more common in men and seldom appears before the age of 50. The motor neurons degenerate until their function is destroyed. When the upper part of the spine is involved, there is difficulty in swallowing and speaking, with weakness of the tongue, throat, and voice box. Food may enter the lungs and cause infection, the vocal cords are paralyzed, and the person cannot cough. The muscles of respiration gradually weaken so that unassisted breathing becomes impossible.

The pure lower motor neuron types of the disease are much less severe than amyotrophic lateral sclerosis. They include conditions formerly known as spinal muscular atrophy and progressive muscular atrophy, and they vary in terms of the age of onset. They usually start with wasting and weakness of the muscles of one limb, affecting the hand or foot and progressing until the affected limb becomes useless.

Amyotrophic lateral sclerosis is usually fatal. Death often results, within two years, from an inability to breathe, choking, or pneumonia owing to the inhalation of food. Death may also be due to malnutrition, because of difficulties swallowing.

The outlook in cases of lower motor neuron disease varies with the different forms. The recessive genetic adult form starts at any age from 15 to 60 but usually begins in the forties. Limb weakness and serious difficulty with walking seldom occur until the sixties or seventies.

SEE ALSO

MUSCLE • MUSCLE DISEASES AND DISORDERS • NERVOUS SYSTEM • PHYSICAL THERAPY • SPINAL CORD

Muscle

All the movements of the body, from the simple twitch of an eyebrow to performing a high jump, are made possible by the muscles. There are three different kinds of muscles: voluntary, involuntary, and cardiac.

Voluntary muscles are under the conscious control of the brain. They are the muscles that are used when a person decides to carry out an action, such as raising an arm, turning the page of a book, smiling, or frowning. This type of muscle is also called striated (striped) muscle, because it looks striped under a microscope. Voluntary muscles are attached to the bones by ligaments and work in pairs to move the bones. Signals from the brain are carried to the muscles by nerves. When a person wants to raise an arm, for example, chemicals are released that make one muscle contract and pull up the arm. The other muscle of the pair relaxes. Voluntary muscles are often subject to injury, but they can self-repair. Sometimes, if one muscle has been damaged, another muscle will grow larger to compensate for the weakened muscle.

Involuntary muscles control all the things that the body does automatically and unconsciously, such as the working of the digestive system and the bladder. They are also called smooth muscles, because they appear unstriped under a microscope. They contract slowly and rhythmically. These muscles may be stimulated by nerves, but some of the chemicals in the body, called hormones, can also control them.

Cardiac muscles make up the main bulk of the heart. Under a

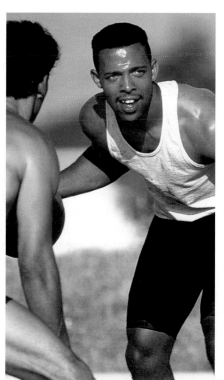

A basketball player uses hundreds of voluntary muscles, unconscious of the hard work being done by his involuntary muscles and heart muscle. Good muscle tone and strength are achieved through regular training.

microscope, they look similar to voluntary muscles. They are controlled by a regulating device in the heart itself, and there is no conscious control over this kind of muscle.

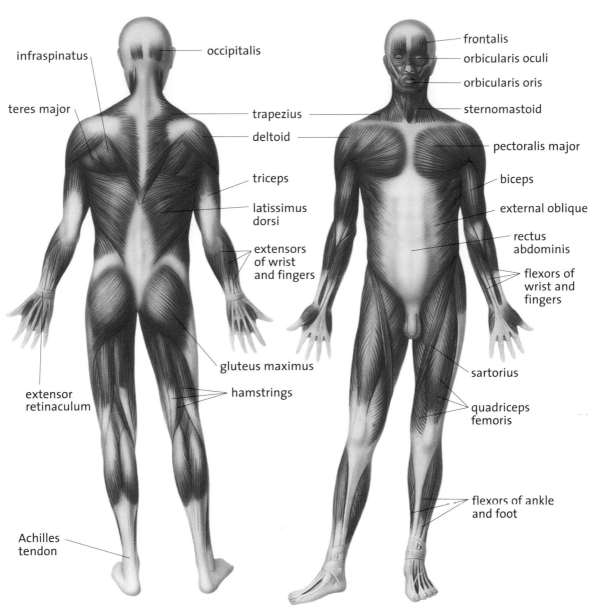

infraspinatus

teres major

occipitalis

trapezius

deltoid

triceps

latissimus dorsi

extensors of wrist and fingers

gluteus maximus

hamstrings

extensor retinaculum

Achilles tendon

frontalis

orbicularis oculi

orbicularis oris

sternomastoid

pectoralis major

biceps

external oblique

rectus abdominis

flexors of wrist and fingers

sartorius

quadriceps femoris

flexors of ankle and foot

These diagrams show front and back views of some of the main voluntary muscles that are located throughout the body.

SEE ALSO

BODY SYSTEMS • HEART • MUSCLE DISEASES AND DISORDERS • REFLEXES • SPORTS INJURIES • SPRAINS AND STRAINS

Muscle Diseases and Disorders

The most common muscle problems are caused by injuries, which often happen to people who take part in active sports. Pulled, strained, and torn muscles are all the same type of injury.

Muscle injuries

Tearing of the muscle fibers and bleeding inside the muscle cause pain and swelling. This kind of injury usually heals quickly, particularly in young people. Treatment usually consists of resting the muscle as much as possible to give it time to knit together and bandaging it for support. When the pain and swelling have gone down, the muscle can gradually be exercised back into use. If any injury remains swollen and painful for more than a few days, a doctor should be consulted.

Sometimes, the whole muscle is torn, or ruptured. This condition is extremely painful, and the muscle will need to be stitched together again. Occasionally, a torn muscle causes bleeding in the muscle and the formation of a blood clot, which is removed surgically.

Muscle cramps and myositis

A cramp is the painful tightening of a muscle or group of muscles. It occurs most commonly in the leg muscles, particularly in the calf. A cramp can come on suddenly, sometimes when a person is asleep. The muscle fibers contract into a hard knot during the spasm, which can last from a few seconds up to a couple of minutes. A cramp can be caused by poor circulation and by exposure to cold. Heavy sweating due to vigorous exercise in a hot climate can deplete the body of salt, causing a cramp. Young people and others engaging in sports should avoid eating just before physical exertion, because the blood is concentrated around the intestines and away from the muscles during digestion, so a cramp may result. Swimmers are particularly at risk. An attack of cramp can be eased by massaging the affected muscle. Flexing the foot upward or manually lifting the toes helps to relieve leg and foot cramp.

Inflammation of the muscle sheaths is known as myositis. It can be caused by cold, by excess exercise, or by an

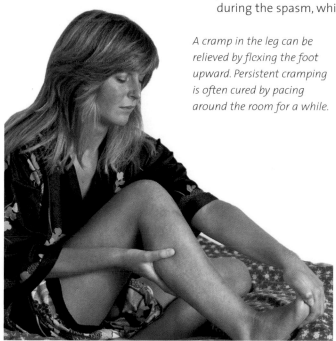

A cramp in the leg can be relieved by flexing the foot upward. Persistent cramping is often cured by pacing around the room for a while.

MUSCLE DISORDERS

Disorder	Causes	Symptoms	Treatments
Pulls, tears, strains, and sprains	Tearing of the muscle fibers, followed by bleeding in and swelling of the affected muscle	Pain, which may become worse during the first few days after original injury; limited movement	Cold (ice packs, water) and pressure with bandages help immediately; later, gentle muscle movement; heat treatment may help
Cramp	Muscle goes into spasm; dehydration may be a cause	Painful tightening of the muscles, often in the calf	Quinine may help; salt and water replacement are vital when dehydration is the cause
Polymyalgia rheumatica	Inflammation of the blood vessels supplying blood to the muscles	Pain, often around the neck and shoulders, and ill-health; affects only the elderly	Anti-inflammatory drugs
Myositis	Painful inflammation of the muscles, often with associated conditions; can be caused by infection	Pain and weakness; blood tests may show that muscle tissue is being broken down	Treatment depends on the cause; rest alone will improve many types, but steroid tablets may help
Muscular dystrophy	Inherited abnormalities in the working of muscle cells	Progressive weakness of muscles affecting different areas according to the form of muscular dystrophy	None, but splints and other aids can be of considerable value
Hypokalemic paralysis	Low level of potassium in blood	Periodic attacks of paralysis	Requires expert medical attention
Hyperkalemic paralysis	High level of potassium in blood	Periodic attacks of paralysis	Requires expert medical attention

PULLED MUSCLES

A muscle can be pulled, strained, or overstretched in an accident or during exercise. The main symptom is pain. The type of injury varies. For example, dropping a heavy load can cause a sudden, sharp movement or moment of acute tension in a particular muscle. Attempting to lift something that is too heavy, or lifting awkwardly or incorrectly, can also cause a pulled muscle. A powerful movement that twists a part of the body into an unnatural position, as often occurs in basketball, may also stretch muscles beyond their natural limit.

infection. Rubbing the area with liniment and taking mild painkillers can ease the pain.

Causes of diseases and disorders

Diseases affecting the muscles are relatively rare. Most muscle weaknesses are caused indirectly: for example, by a problem occurring in the nervous system, which controls the movement of the muscles. Lou Gehrig's disease is this type of disorder or motor neuron disease. Occasionally, a hormonal condition or a lack of vitamin D can result in a weakening of the muscles. Other serious muscle disorders, such as muscular dystrophy, are inherited.

SEE ALSO

ANALGESICS • CRAMPS • EXERCISE • MOTOR NEURON DISEASE • MUSCLE • NERVOUS SYSTEM • PAIN • SPORTS INJURIES • SPRAINS AND STRAINS • VITAMINS

Nervous System

The nervous system is the body's complex communications and control network. It collects information around the body through the senses of sight, hearing, taste, smell, and touch, and then it tells the body what to do in response. The nervous system consists of millions of interconnected nerve cells called neurons; they pick up information and send signals from one part of the system to another. Neurons are easily damaged or destroyed by injury, infection, pressure, chemical disturbance, or lack of oxygen.

The nervous system consists of the peripheral nervous system and the central nervous system. The central nervous system consists of the brain and the spinal cord. Together they receive messages from the body's sense organs, analyze them, and then send out signals to the muscles and glands. Thousands of neurons are involved in the brain during this assessment. The peripheral nervous system consists of all the nerve tissue outside the central nervous system. Nerves branch out from the brain and spinal cord and then divide to supply the body. The peripheral nervous system consists of an outer system (the somatic or body system) and an inner one (the autonomic system).

The somatic system collects information from the body's sense organs and conveys it to the central nervous system along sensory nerve fibers. It carries signals from the central nervous system to the muscles along motor nerve fibers, which are gathered into a bundle called a nerve. Forty-three pairs of nerves emerge from the central nervous system. Twelve pairs come from the brain; the rest of them come from the spinal cord.

The autonomic nervous system controls unconscious functions, such as the heartbeat, the narrowing and widening of blood vessels, breathing, and gland secretion. Autonomic control becomes extremely active in times of sudden physical danger and modifies body function to give the body the best chance of survival.

Each neuron has the same basic structure, but neurons are of various shapes and sizes. Each neuron cell has a number of fine, rootlike fibers, or dendrites, projecting from it. Projecting from the cell is a single, long fiber called an axon. At its far end, the axon either ends in a single tiny knob or divides into a number of branches, ending in a cluster of knobs. Each knob is separated by a minute gap from a dendrite, from another neuron, or from the surface of a muscle cell or a gland cell. Messages are carried across these gaps by substances called neurotransmitters. Every neuron has a thin wall known as the neural membrane, which is vital for the transmission of signals. Many axons have an insulating covering called myelin.

Q & A

A friend said the pain I have in my hands and arms could be caused by a pinched nerve. What is this?

At some point along their length, many nerves have to pass through a restricted space, especially near joints. Any displacement or swelling in this space may squeeze or pinch the nerve, causing pain, muscle weakness, numbness, or a tingling sensation.

Two months ago, my grandfather had a foot amputated. I'm extremely confused because he still feels that the foot is there and even has pain from the missing toes. Why does this happen?

Although his foot has been amputated, the sensory fibers that used to send messages from the foot to the brain are still present in the remaining part of his leg and have their endings in the stump. If these endings are stimulated, the fibers send messages via the spinal cord to the brain, which, from past experience, interprets the message as having come from the foot.

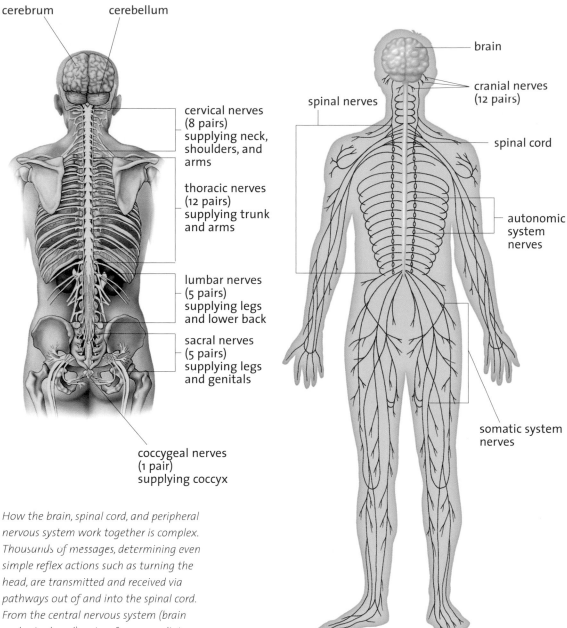

cerebrum

cerebellum

cervical nerves
(8 pairs)
supplying neck,
shoulders, and
arms

thoracic nerves
(12 pairs)
supplying trunk
and arms

lumbar nerves
(5 pairs)
supplying legs
and lower back

sacral nerves
(5 pairs)
supplying legs
and genitals

coccygeal nerves
(1 pair)
supplying coccyx

brain

cranial nerves
(12 pairs)

spinal nerves

spinal cord

autonomic
system
nerves

somatic system
nerves

How the brain, spinal cord, and peripheral nervous system work together is complex. Thousands of messages, determining even simple reflex actions such as turning the head, are transmitted and received via pathways out of and into the spinal cord. From the central nervous system (brain and spinal cord), pairs of nerves radiate all over the body, forming the peripheral system. This system has two main subdivisions: the autonomic system (unconscious control of functions such as breathing) and the somatic system (conscious control).

SEE ALSO

BODY SYSTEMS • MOTOR NEURON DISEASE • PAIN • SPINAL
COLUMN • SPINAL CORD

Nosebleed

Q & A

I've heard that a nosebleed is a sign of pressure on the brain. My brother has had several nosebleeds recently. Is this serious?

Nosebleeds are common in children, perhaps because they are so active and thus are likely to have many minor injuries. Some children are more prone to nosebleeds than others. A frequent cause is that blood vessels just inside one or both nostrils have burst, after becoming weakened and enlarged through rubbing and picking, or because of previous nosebleeds. Pressure on the brain is not a cause. However, recurrent bleeding can be a symptom of disease, so your parents should consult your brother's doctor.

My grandmother used to put a cloth soaked in witch hazel across my nose when it bled. Is this an effective cure?

Although some herbs may have properties that help stem the flow of blood, it is more likely that your grandmother's treatment acted as an effective cold compress.

A nosebleed is caused by the breaking of a small blood vessel inside the nose. It may be the result of direct violence, injury, sneezing, or picking the nose. Some people have a nosebleed when they have an attack of hay fever or have a nasal infection. If the membranes lining the nose become dry and cracked, bleeding may occur. Sometimes, there is no obvious reason for it. Girls who have recently started to menstruate often have nosebleeds with no apparent cause.

A broken nose, one of the most common sports injuries, often results in a nosebleed and requires immediate medical attention. Almost invariably, a broken nose will be out of shape. If it is allowed to heal without being reset by a surgeon, it will lead in most cases to other problems, such as chronic runny nose or sinusitis (inflammation of a sinus).

First aid for a nosebleed

The person with a nosebleed should sit quietly, loosen the clothes around the neck, and lean his or her head slightly forward (not back) to help prevent any blood from being swallowed. He or she should pinch together the nostrils until the bleeding stops, while breathing gently through the mouth. If bleeding continues, a small, clean piece of gauze should be inserted just inside one or both nostrils, which should then be pressed together. It is important not to force anything up the nose. When the bleeding stops, it is important that the patient does not keep touching the nose. If bleeding does not stop, a doctor should be consulted or the patient should be taken to a hospital.

Serious nosebleeds

Sometimes, an artery at the back of the nose is damaged, causing extremely heavy bleeding. That situation needs treatment by a doctor, who will pack the nose. Other nosebleeds also need attention from a doctor: those caused by a blow, those that happen within a week or so of a tonsil or adenoid operation, and those lasting for more than about 20 minutes. Otherwise, home treatment is usually sufficient.

Although nosebleeds can often be alarming, not much blood is lost, even during a heavy nosebleed. Normally, a nosebleed clears up in five to 15 minutes, which is the time it usually takes for blood to clot.

SEE ALSO

CIRCULATORY SYSTEM • ICE THERAPY • SPORTS INJURIES

Nutritional Diseases

The body can work properly only if it receives the right materials, including certain vitamins and minerals. Without them, people develop diseases such as scurvy and rickets. In the past, although it was known how to prevent certain diseases, it was not known what the causes were. Experts are now learning more about the substances the body needs. In developed countries, few people suffer from deficiency diseases. However, in some countries in the developing world where people have an inadequate diet, there is a serious problem.

Sometimes, people do not eat properly because they cannot get enough food. Others do not know what to eat or do not eat sensibly. Alcoholics often get deficiency diseases, for example, because they do not eat properly and do not absorb fats and vitamins. Beriberi (degenerative changes of the nerves, digestive system, and the heart) is caused by lack of vitamin B_1 (thiamine). However, most deficiency diseases are easy to cure with a proper diet. The diet may be supplemented with large doses of the substance that has been lacking.

A few people have nutritional diseases even though they are eating properly, because their bodies are unable to take in or use certain substances properly. For example, some people become anemic because their bodies cannot absorb vitamin B_{12}. If people eat sensibly, they should get everything they need from their food. Vitamin and mineral supplements should be taken only if a doctor prescribes them, because too many vitamins can be harmful.

CONDITIONS CAUSED BY NUTRITIONAL DEFICIENCY

VITAMIN OR MINERAL DEFICIENCY	DISEASES AND DISORDERS	DEFICIENCY CORRECTED BY
Vitamin A	Skin diseases, severe conjunctivitis, night blindness	Dairy products, eggs, liver, oily fish, vegetables (especially carrots)
Vitamin B_1 (thiamine)	Beriberi (weakness, swelling), confusion, heart failure	Bran, cereals, pork, liver
Vitamin B (niacin)	Pellagra (a skin disorder), diarrhea, dementia, dermatitis with skin blistering	Liver, kidney, yeast, fish, cereals
Vitamin C	Scurvy, slow wound healing, anemia, hemorrhages from tooth sockets and into joints	Fresh fruits and vegetables
Vitamin D	Disorders of bone formation leading to swelling, softening, and bowing of bones (called osteomalacia in adults and rickets in children)	Milk, egg yolk, cod liver oil, fortified milk and margarine, action of sunlight on skin
Iron	Anemia	Lean meat, liver, spinach, cabbage, legumes, eggs
Sodium	Disturbances of body chemistry	Salt
Iodine	Goiter (swelling of thyroid gland), cretinism	Seafood

SEE ALSO

ANEMIA · CALCIUM · DIET · DIGESTIVE SYSTEM · FOOD AND NUTRITION · IODINE · IRON · MALNUTRITION · MILK · MINERALS · PROTEIN · SALT · SCURVY · VITAMINS

Obesity

If the amount of food people eat exceeds the energy used, they will become overweight. If a person's weight is 20 percent or more above normal for his or her height and age, there will be an accumulation of body fat and the person will be obese. Obesity can be prevented by sensible eating and by exercise. It can be cured by dieting and then eating carefully. This is not easy, but it is worth doing. Obesity is a serious condition, because it increases the risk of developing various chronic health problems.

Causes

The amount of food someone's body uses varies a great deal from one person to another, but if a person is gaining weight, he or she is eating more than is needed. The excess food is converted into fat that is stored under the skin, first in cells in the buttocks and around the waist, and later in the thighs, shoulders, and arms. Very rarely, a medical problem such as an underactive thyroid gland causes obesity by greatly reducing energy expenditure. Medical tests will find out if there is any such cause. Bad eating habits are the most common cause of obesity. Often, all the members of a family are obese, because they have similar habits. Emotional problems can make people overeat for comfort.

Dangers and treatments

Extra weight puts strain on the joints, particularly the knees, hips, and some of the back joints. It causes wear and tear, which may become a painful problem. Someone with a very fat stomach cannot breathe properly, and he or she will have shortness of breath and lung problems. Obesity can cause gallstones; mild

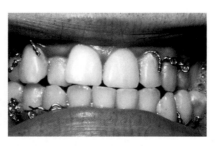

diabetes, in turn causing serious complications in the small blood vessels of the eyes and kidneys; thickening of the arteries, which increases the likelihood of suffering a stroke or heart attack; and high blood pressure.

SEE ALSO

ANOREXIA AND BULIMIA • BLOOD PRESSURE • CALORIES • CIRCULATORY SYSTEM • DIABETES • DIET • DIETING • EXERCISE • FOOD AND NUTRITION • GLANDS • HEART • HEART ATTACK • HIP • ISOMETRIC EXERCISES • JOINT DISORDERS • JOINTS • KNEE • SPORTS • STROKE • WEIGHT CONTROL

Q & A

My friend eats the same amount as I do, is about the same height as I am, but is of average weight, whereas I am fat. Why is this?

The way in which people's bodies use food varies widely. People who use their food fuel economically become obese more easily than those who use it extravagantly, because they burn off less energy for the same amount of work. You may also find that you are getting less exercise than your friend, so that you are expending less energy. Finally, you may have acquired an excess of fat as a child, so that even if you eat the same as your friend, you are still not losing your excess stored fat.

Is it true that gland trouble can cause obesity?

People are rarely overweight because of an underactive thyroid gland or overactive adrenal glands, and in these cases, there are other symptoms.

This woman has resorted to desperate measures to help reduce her weight. She has had her teeth wired so that her jaws are clamped together. She can consume liquids only.

Orthopedics

The term *orthopedics* derives from the Greek root *ortho*, meaning "straight." Orthopedics is the surgical specialty that is concerned with disorders and deformities of the bones, joints, ligaments, muscles, and tendons. The specialty is also concerned with nerves that are involved in skeletal injuries or in conditions leading to muscle weakness. Orthopedics covers many disorders involving these body systems. Some disorders are present at birth (congenital) and some are acquired later in life. They may be inflammatory and due to infection; degenerative or the result of tumors; or, in many cases, due to injury. An important part of orthopedics is the treatment of the complications of the various forms of arthritis.

Fractures and other bone disorders

Orthopedic surgeons treat difficult fractures, especially when recovery is delayed or complicated by soft-tissue injuries, or when the break is adjacent to nerves and blood vessels. Most fractures heal satisfactorily if the limb is immobilized with a plaster cast or by other means. However, if healing is hindered, orthopedic help is needed. Some fractures are so fragmented that they cannot be kept in alignment or immobilized by an external cast. Sometimes, there is damage to blood or nerve supplies. Compound fractures (those that involve open wounds) need treatment by a specialist. In some cases, fractures that have not united need bone grafting. Orthopedic surgery can involve fixing a fracture with screws, plates, or nails inside the bone.

Orthopedists are also concerned with other bone disorders, including bone growth failure, bone softening, bone distortion from rickets in children or from osteomalacia in older people, bone tumors, and tuberculosis of the bone. Degenerative bone diseases and congenital defects of the skeleton require careful

Q & A

My brother had an accident recently and is in a body cast. Will his skin suffer?

The skin grows even when it is covered by a plaster cast. When the plaster is finally removed, the skin will look dirty and have the appearance of sandpaper, because it has continued to grow and has shed scales. This is not a long-term problem and should improve within a few weeks.

When a person breaks a bone, is it best to have a bone graft or to have a pin inserted?

It is always better to let things heal naturally whenever possible. A pin, a plate, or another piece of metal is used in the join only if the orthopedic surgeon believes the fracture will not unite firmly without it. A pin holds two bones together; a graft adds bone pieces that are missing. A cast keeps the injury immobile during the healing process.

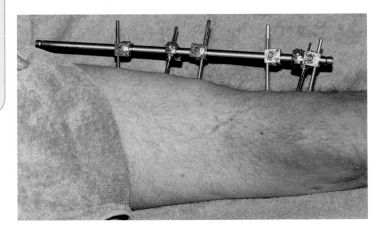

If a bone is fractured in several places, external pins may be used to immobilize and fix the bone. The pins are inserted through the skin into the bone and are held in place externally with a metal rod.

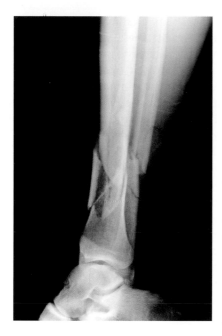

This X-ray shows a spiral comminuted fracture of the tibia and fibula, which are the bones of the lower leg. In this type of fracture, the bone is broken, splintered, or crushed into a number of pieces and will require orthopedic treatment.

management. One advance in orthopedics is the use of bone-lengthening procedures to treat certain forms of dwarfism. With a growing elderly population, the incidence of osteoporosis in women after menopause is becoming increasingly high. Osteoporosis can make bones so brittle that they break easily. Spinal bone problems in older women are usually due to osteoporosis. Fractures of the neck of the femur are also common in women with osteoporosis. The blood supply to the head of the bone may be cut off when the femoral neck is fractured. That can lead to the need for an artificial hip replacement, which is one of the most common operations performed by orthopedic surgeons.

Joint injuries and foot conditions

Joint injuries are common and range from simple sprains, in which some of the ligaments are slightly stretched, to radical dislocations with extensive soft-tissue damage. Some joints, such as the shoulder joint, are liable to recurrent dislocations that require surgery. Other common orthopedic problems are joint disorders of the knee from twisting injuries or direct force, in which the cartilage of the knee joint is torn and displaced, with locking of the joint. The internal ligaments, which stabilize the joint, may be stretched or torn. Various surgeries are done on the interior of the knee joint with an arthroscope, a fine instrument that is passed into the joint through a tiny incision that allows illumination and visualization, and the use of specially designed surgical instruments. Tears of external knee ligaments may be repaired by open surgery.

The joint between the big toe and the first long bone of the foot (metatarsal) is commonly distorted by a genetic tendency or by unsuitable shoes to form a bunion, a bony bulge with overlying soft tissue. In severe cases, the only treatment is to chisel off the bony bulge. Other orthopedic foot conditions include congenital clubfoot (talipes), flatfoot, and hammertoe (in which a toe is fixed in an angular position). Inflammatory disorders of joints are common and can be hard to treat. Some, such as gout, can be treated medically and do not involve orthopedics. In many cases, however, orthopedic surgery is invaluable in restoring comfort and function by joint replacement.

SEE ALSO

ARTHRITIS • FRACTURES AND DISLOCATIONS • JOINTS • KNEE • LIGAMENTS • MUSCLE • MUSCLE DISEASES AND DISORDERS • SHOULDER • SKELETAL SYSTEM • SKIN • SPRAINS AND STRAINS

Osteopathy

Osteopathy is a system of diagnosis and treatment that recognizes the role of the muscles and skeletal system in the healthy functioning of the body. An osteopath is a medical practitioner who has graduated from an osteopathic medical school and holds a doctorate in osteopathic medicine (DO).

Osteopaths stress the importance of the correct functioning and position of the bones, the muscles, and their connecting tendons and ligaments in general health. They concentrate on musculoskeletal manipulation and take a distinctly holistic (whole-person) approach to consultation, diagnosis, and practice. Osteopathy also focuses on promoting wellness, rather than simply treating the symptoms of a disease.

Osteopathic treatment includes manipulating the bones, muscles, and joints to relieve pain and discomfort, improve mobility, and restore body control mechanisms. Most people visit osteopaths because they have sports injuries, back pain, or restricted movement in a joint. An osteopath is usually able to treat patients successfully using a combination of manipulation, rhythmic stretching, and pressure.

Q & A

Are chiropractors and osteopaths the same?

No. Chiropractors practice only musculoskeletal manipulations. Osteopaths may do some manipulation, but they are fully trained and qualified physicians who can prescribe medicines, whereas chiropractors cannot.

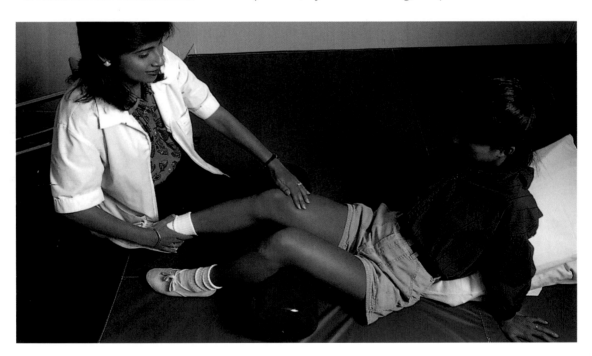

Osteopathic treatment begins with a thorough examination of the patient. The osteopath then decides what type of manipulative treatment to apply.

SEE ALSO

CHIROPRACTIC • JOINT DISORDERS • JOINTS • LIGAMENTS • MUSCLE • SKELETAL SYSTEM • SPORTS INJURIES • TENDON

Oxygen

Q & A

My grandfather is in the hospital and has to have oxygen. Will he always need this extra supply of oxygen?

No; he is unlikely to need extra oxygen when he leaves the hospital. The usual reason people are given oxygen in the hospital is that they have an acute heart problem or an infection in the chest when they already suffer from a long-term chest ailment. The extra oxygen helps them with the immediate difficulty, and it is controlled very carefully.

I often feel tired and lethargic. Am I short of oxygen?

No, probably not. Everybody feels tired sometimes, but oxygen shortage is rarely the cause. Some heart or lung conditions can make a person breathless with exercise. Anemia, however, can cause a person to become tired and listless and involves a low oxygen level. Consult your doctor if you are worried.

Green plants give off oxygen, which is breathed in by humans and other animals; they breathe out carbon dioxide, which is taken in and used by the plants. This is known as the oxygen cycle.

Oxygen is a gas, with no smell, taste, or color. It makes up about one-fifth of the air that people and other animals breathe. Oxygen is an important substance on which many forms of life depend.

People cannot live for more than a few minutes without oxygen, because it is essential for producing energy. The main task of the lungs, heart, and blood vessels is to carry oxygen from the air to every part of the body. The brain, in particular, requires a large, continuous supply of oxygen. Deprivation of oxygen for more than a few minutes usually produces serious brain damage and is often fatal.

A shortage of oxygen in the body shows up as a blueness around the lips and tongue, a condition known as cyanosis. People most likely to suffer from a shortage of oxygen are those with lung disease, including chronic bronchitis, acute attacks of asthma, pneumonia, and emphysema.

Heart complaints that keep the lungs short of blood can cause oxygen starvation, and patients have to be given extra oxygen through a mask.

Oxygen therapy

Oxygen is by far the most vital element for human life and health. Failure to get an adequate supply of oxygen to the body's tissues causes a range of diseases in which the intake of oxygen to the blood or the supply of blood to the tissues is reduced. Oxygen therapy is often an essential part of medical treatment.

Hyperbaric (high-pressure) oxygen therapy provides a massive

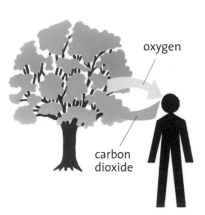

oxygen

carbon dioxide

supply of oxygen to the patient's tissues. This is necessary in heart surgery and is helpful in treating carbon monoxide poisoning, decompression sickness, and nonhealing wounds. Infections that function only in the absence of oxygen, such as tetanus and gas gangrene, can also be treated with oxygen.

SEE ALSO

ANEMIA • ASTHMA • CIRCULATORY SYSTEM • HEART • HEART ATTACK • LETHARGY • RESPIRATORY SYSTEM • TIREDNESS

Pain

Pain is the body's alarm system. It acts as a warning when something is wrong. Pain should never be ignored; neither should people keep taking painkillers to blot out pain if they do not know what is causing it. A doctor should be able to find out why the pain exists and provide the treatment needed to cure it.

Causes of pain

Pain is caused by something stimulating the tiny nerve ends that are present in all parts of the body. Sometimes, pain produces an instant reaction. If a person touches something very hot, the body will draw back the hand faster than he or she can think. Sensory nerves have taken the message "hot" to the spinal cord. The motor nerves have acted immediately to remove the hand from the danger. At the same time, nerves are taking messages to the brain, which figures out more slowly what is happening. Internal pains work in the same sort of way.

Types of pains

There are many kinds of pains—from sharp, knifelike pains to dull, throbbing aches. Acute pain is usually intense and short-lived. It may be caused by a burn, a cut, or a blow. Sometimes, acute pain is so severe that the blood vessels dilate, the blood pressure drops, and the person loses consciousness. Chronic pain

Q & A

Why can pain cause a person to faint?

The parts of the brain that receive and analyze painful stimuli have close connections with the parts that have overall control of blood circulation, the heartbeat, and the condition of the peripheral blood vessels. Even a small degree of pain causes some change in a person's pulse rate, blood pressure, or both. If pain is severe, the circulation can be swamped by these influences: the blood vessels dilate and the blood pressure drops so low that unconsciousness results. This process is the same for any severe unpleasant stimulus, although people vary as to what degree of pain causes fainting.

Does acupuncture work only psychologically to relieve pain?

Psychological factors are very important in any method of pain relief, because of the considerable psychological component in the appreciation of pain. However, it is likely that there is a genuine physiological mechanism at work in some methods of acupuncture.

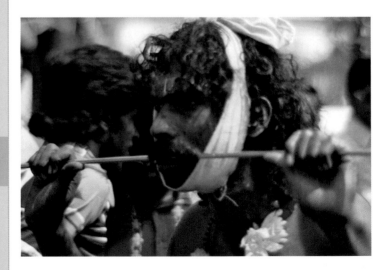

Some cultures make a virtue of pain; this man, taking part in a Hindu religious ceremony, has both cheeks pierced by a metal rod. Like some practitioners of Eastern religions who walk barefoot over red-hot coals, he has a high tolerance of pain. He has trained his mind to ignore painful reactions by concentrating on other—usually spiritually uplifting—things.

is persistent over a relatively long period of time and is invariably the sign of some disorder. It is often characterized by a deep, dull, aching pain. There are many different causes of chronic pain. Sometimes, it is easy to sense where a pain is coming from.

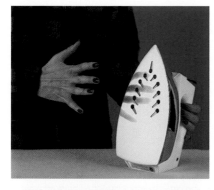

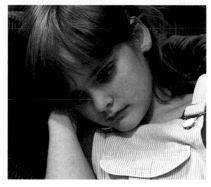

Touching a hot iron (top) causes a sharp pain, followed by a burning sensation. Earache (bottom) may be a dull, persistent pain.

This diagram shows the pathways by which sensations of pain travel to the brain. Analysis of pain begins in the brain stem and goes either directly or on a more meandering course to the thalamus, which is the brain's main sensory relay station.

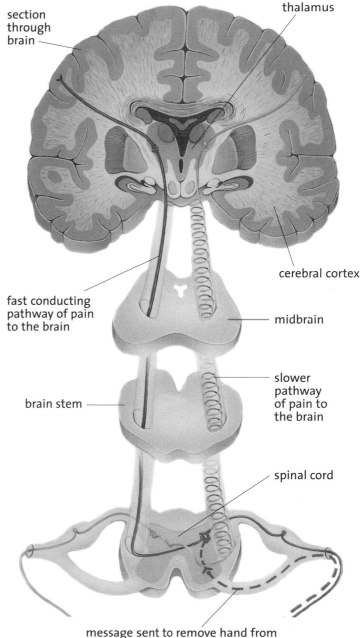

section through brain

thalamus

cerebral cortex

fast conducting pathway of pain to the brain

midbrain

slower pathway of pain to the brain

brain stem

spinal cord

message sent to remove hand from painful stimulus such as hot iron

PAIN RELIEF WITHOUT DRUGS

Transcutaneous electrical nerve stimulation (TENS) is often used for neck and back pain, phantom limb pain, and nerve injury and infection. A tiny portable instrument delivers low-voltage pulses, stimulating nerves that block out the pain. Electrodes are placed on the skin at trigger points, and the instrument is turned on when needed.

Acupuncture is effective for all types of pain, because acupuncture needles stimulate nerves that suppress pain.

Biofeedback machines measure automatic body functions such as muscle tension and brain waves. After training, a person with migraine or tension headaches can recognize the automatic responses that trigger pain; the machines are usually equipped with a warning sound signal. The patient is then able to control the pain by consciously relaxing the muscles or by dilating the blood vessels.

In other cases, pain may seem to come from some general area. To make matters more complicated, pain from some organs of the body may seem to be coming from quite another place. Pain from the heart is felt in the center of the chest and in the left arm and jaw, for example. This is known as referred pain; it occurs because sensory nerves running to a particular segment of the spinal cord may come from widely separated points, and nerve impulses coming from one of these areas may be interpreted as coming from the other.

Phantom limb pain

When an arm or a leg has been amputated, the nerves remain in the stump. If something stimulates their endings, the brain will register the pain as though it were coming from the missing limb. It may take some time before the brain comes to terms with the fact that the limb is no longer there.

Sensitivity to pain

Some people are much more sensitive to pain than others. What is a slight hurt to one person may cause genuinely severe pain to another. A person may also feel a pain much more at one time than at another. In the case of sudden, unexpected severe injury, when pain should be extreme, the injured person may feel little or no pain. In such circumstances, the brain produces morphinelike substances called endorphins, which are highly effective in controlling pain. During a battle, for example, a wounded person may hardly notice his or her injury.

Relieving pain

Analgesics and other drugs are used to control pain. Narcotics such as morphine, codeine, methadone, and meperidine, which are addictive, are used for only a limited time, such as after surgery or a severe injury. There is also a wide range of non-narcotic painkillers. Aspirin and acetaminophen are the most commonly used for minor aches and pains, and prescription analgesics such as propoxyphene may be given by a doctor for certain other types of pain. It is inadvisable to take over-the-counter painkillers for longer than two or three days. If the pain persists, a doctor should be consulted.

SEE ALSO

ACUPRESSURE • ACUPUNCTURE • ANALGESICS • NERVOUS SYSTEM • SPINAL CORD

Paraplegia

Q & A

I have recently been confined to a wheelchair. Should I change my diet?

Yes. You should be eating much less than before. Because you are a lot less active, you will not be able to burn up as many calories; thus you are likely to put on weight, which is not easy to lose when you are confined to a wheelchair.

Paraplegia is damage to the middle or lower area of the spinal cord that can cause paralysis of both legs and sometimes part of the trunk. The connection between the brain and the nerves used for movement is cut. If the damage to the spinal cord is high in the neck, the arms and the legs are also paralyzed, a condition known as tetraplegia or quadriplegia. Most cases of paraplegia involve both legs and the lower part of the trunk.

The most common cause of paraplegia is spinal cord damage from a physical force that fractures and dislocates the spine, compressing or severing the spinal cord. Several small strokes affecting both sides of the brain can also cause paraplegia.

Spinal cord injury can also result from diseases that affect the spinal cord, including myelitis (cord inflammation), multiple sclerosis (MS), poliomyelitis, and blockage by a blood clot in the spinal artery. In children, paraplegia can be caused by congenital malformations of the spinal cord or by early brain damage leading to cerebral palsy. Early rickets, with softening and distortion of the spine, can also cause cord damage and paraplegia.

The degree of damage to the cord determines the degree of sensation that is lost. In some cases, there is paralysis and loss of sensation in the entire body below the level of the injury. In addition to the inability to walk, paraplegia often causes problems with bladder and bowel control.

Much research is now under way to find ways to rejoin nerves. Already, paraplegia has been cured in small animals, and experts are optimistic. In addition, a frame that allows a paraplegic to walk has been designed. The frame has leg braces and splints and is assisted by the arms and by electric motors. Improvements in the design are being made constantly.

Electrical stimulation of the paralyzed leg muscles to make them contract and allow a paraplegic to walk are also being developed.

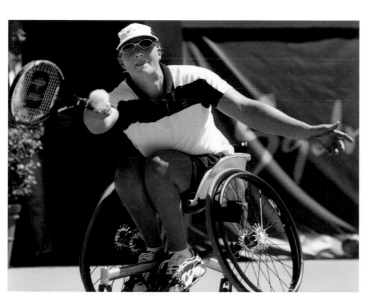

Paraplegia does not prevent people from playing competitive sports. Esther Vergeer of the Netherlands is seen here playing in the paralympics in Sydney, Australia, in 2000.

> **SEE ALSO**
>
> LEG • MUSCLE • NERVOUS SYSTEM • SPINAL COLUMN • SPINAL CORD • SPORTS • STROKE

Physical Examination

Q & A

Most of the time, I just don't feel very good. Should I ask my doctor to give me a thorough physical examination?

If you feel bad for any length of time, it is important that you go to your doctor to find out what is wrong. Normally, he or she will be able to assure you that there is nothing wrong. However, if there is any doubt, the doctor will probably recommend a full physical examination.

Someone told me that all children should have an annual physical examination. Is this right?

It is certainly wise for children to have regular medical and dental checkups to make sure that they are developing normally and that there are no signs of disease. It is not usually necessary, however, for these to be done as often as once a year. It is desirable that adolescents have a checkup twice a year during their time of most rapid growth.

A physical examination is usually a part of a consultation with a physician. Generally, only the area of the body that is affected will be examined, but on occasion, the doctor will give the patient a thorough examination. Children and teenagers should have several physical examinations during their growing period. Many companies insist that their key employees have regular checkups. Such examinations can detect the onset of disease before any symptoms appear.

A typical physical examination would include palpating (feeling) the abdomen and other parts to discover any tenderness or swelling. The doctor also percusses (taps) the chest and abdomen to detect whether there are areas of unexpected dullness or resonance. The doctor listens through a stethoscope to sound-producing organs such as the heart and lungs. Other tests may include measuring blood pressure, having a laboratory analyze urine and blood, taking X-rays, and perhaps taking an electrocardiogram.

In 1987, the American Heart Association recommended that, to detect and prevent heart and blood disease, everybody should have regular checkups every five years from the age of 20. After people reach 65, the checkups should be every two and a half years. At age 75, the examinations should be done every year.

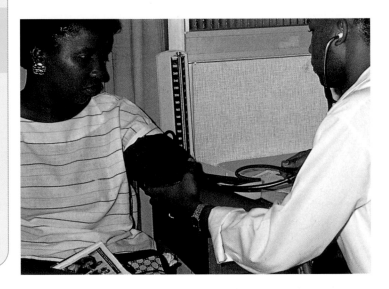

This woman is having her blood pressure checked. High blood pressure can be extremely dangerous; low blood pressure can signal inadequate blood flow to various parts of the body.

SEE ALSO

AGING • BLOOD PRESSURE • BODY SYSTEMS • CHOLESTEROL • GROWTH • PHYSICAL FITNESS • PUBERTY

Physical Fitness

Physical fitness is not simply exercise. It means getting and keeping the body in a condition that will maintain good health, while developing physical endurance and skill so that life can be enjoyed to the fullest through functioning at the best physical level. Physical fitness involves a healthy, balanced diet, which is necessary to fuel the body and its muscles properly.

To achieve physical fitness, people also need to have the right mental attitude. If they recognize the health benefits of physical fitness, they must be willing to put in the effort to build up stamina and endurance in the sports, exercise programs, and fitness activities they most enjoy.

Benefits of physical fitness

The benefits of physical fitness are that a person looks and feels better and the ordinary everyday tasks of life are easy. A sound body also helps the brain use energy efficiently so that concentration and learning become easier.

Physical activity can also clear the mind of stress and depression, leaving people feeling refreshed and invigorated. As a lifelong benefit, physical fitness may help people live longer by preventing or delaying the onset of some diseases.

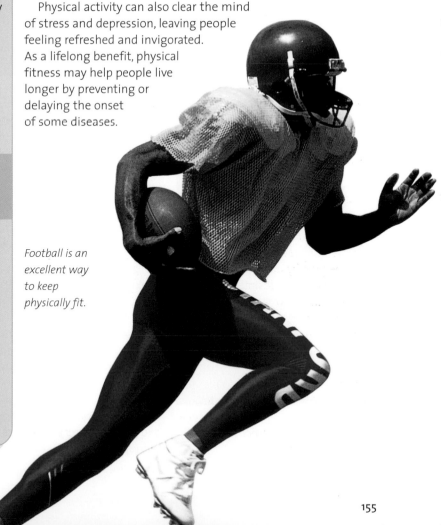

Football is an excellent way to keep physically fit.

Q & A

How quickly will my body adapt itself to my new fitness regimen? At the moment, I ache all over.

You may be doing too much too soon; slow down a bit. As you get fitter, you will be able to do more without feeling such ill effects. Your body has probably been underused for a long time; do not expect it to be in prime condition after only a few days or weeks. There should not be too much suffering involved in getting fit; more discomfort should be felt during exercise than afterward.

Are all children naturally physically fit or do they have to work at fitness?

The younger children are, the less they have to work at their physical fitness. As they grow older, however, the situation changes; there will be a noticeable difference between the performance of teenage athletes and their untrained friends. People from their twenties onward definitely need regular exercise for real fitness. Whatever one's age, it is important to maintain fitness.

Basketball is the most popular sport in high schools in the United States. It helps build muscles and is good for overall conditioning, because of its relatively high aerobic value.

THE RIGHT CLOTHING

Loose, comfortable clothing that will not restrict movement should be worn during exercising. Tight jeans and tops inhibit movement. Warm clothing is needed in cold weather to prevent tight, sore muscles and cramps. Layers of clothing are best to soak up sweat. For joggers and runners, good sneakers are vital. For skiers, good skis with efficient bindings and automatic release in a fall are essential.

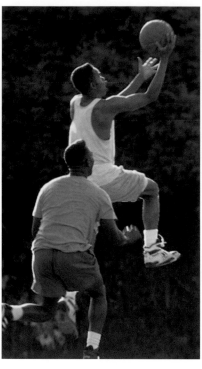

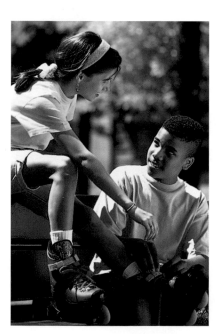

Rollerblading is a good form of exercise that can be enjoyed outdoors.

Lifestyle and physical fitness

Increasing numbers of people are now concerned about physical fitness, and many individuals participate in sports and physical activities as a matter of routine. Often, whole families jog together, and jogging is one of the best activities for overall fitness. However, many people frequently embark on a fitness program and then give it up after a few weeks. One reason is that they fail to realize that the commitment to fitness is a lifelong contract between themselves and their bodies. They must be prepared to persist so that physical activity becomes a habit and an enjoyable and fulfilling part of everyday life.

The first step is to choose enjoyable activities that fit easily into one's lifestyle. Jogging or cycling to school, for example, may take only half an hour longer than the bus, but students will start the school day feeling much more invigorated. Dancing for a couple of hours a week is another vigorous and healthy exercise that is happily and easily accommodated in people's lifestyle, whatever their age.

Developing lifelong habits

At school, students should participate in sports that they enjoy, but they should remember that fitness for specific sports does not necessarily mean overall fitness. Some activities, such as gymnastics and karate, help muscular development and flexibility but do not fully exercise the heart and lungs in the same way as aerobics does. Basketball and racquetball have a relatively high aerobic value, but many young people give up these sports after high school or college. Unless they take up another activity, they lapse into unfitness. It is a good idea to take up a lifelong sport, such as swimming or tennis, as part of one's training and conditioning.

EXERCISE SAFETY CODE

- Always warm up for 15 to 20 minutes with basic calisthenics or stretching exercises.
- Stop when you are tired, and before you are exhausted.
- Stop if you are in pain.
- Stop if you feel dizzy or nauseated.
- Take your pulse regularly.
- Never exercise if you have a fever or viral infection.
- Always wear suitable clothing for the type of exercise or sport.
- Always cool down afterward to relax and allow the pulse rate to return to normal.

Achieving maximum physical fitness

To achieve maximum physical fitness, a combination of aerobic exercise and isotonic exercise should be undertaken. Aerobic exercise increases the amount of oxygen in the blood and provides an improved oxygen supply to the body's tissues, helping create a stronger heart and healthier lungs. Isotonic exercises develop muscular strength and flexibility. Aerobic exercise causes breathlessness, but if it is a regular activity, as performance time increases, so does the time before breathlessness starts. Cycling, running, swimming, and jogging are excellent aerobic activities.

Rowing, gymnastics, and skiing are sports with high isotonic value, as are exercise programs that include stretching, yoga, and weight training. Weight training should not be confused with lifting heavy weights. Weight training involves working out with light weights of only 2 to 5 pounds (1–2 kg) to begin with and then increasing the capacity to lift something a little heavier or for a little longer. Weights help develop strength and endurance and a firmer, leaner-looking body.

When both types of physical activities are combined with a healthy diet and plenty of sleep, peak condition is achieved. People embarking on such a regimen will have few weight problems, will tire less easily, and will feel more relaxed and able to cope with mental activity.

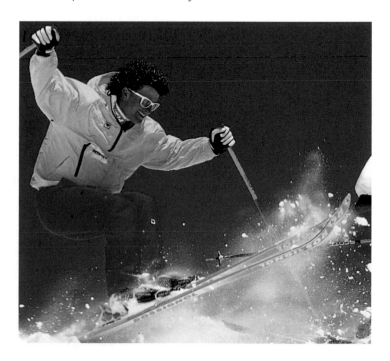

Skiing is an excellent activity for keeping fit, but it is expensive and few people have access to ski slopes all year round.

A wide range of activities

Many young people dislike organized sports and do their best to avoid them. Some have poor eyesight or are overweight. They feel that they cannot compete with their more athletic peers. Others have a disability, such as asthma or diabetes, which limits their activities. For those people who feel they cannot take part in regular fitness programs, there is a wide range of noncompetitive or solo activities that can be fun and easily modified to suit the individual. A good example is swimming, which is a great exercise for all-around fitness. It has high aerobic value, firms and strengthens the muscles of the lower and upper back, and streamlines the whole body. Because water supports body weight, the effort of swimming seems less than it really is.

For asthmatic youngsters, swimming is an ideal activity that helps them breathe more easily. It is important to note that for young diabetics, increased exercise must be balanced with an

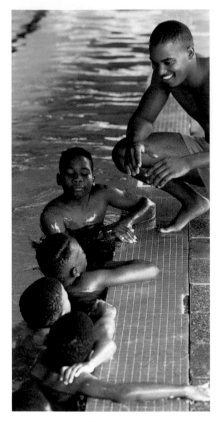

Swimming is the best activity of all for overall fitness. To get the most out of swimming sessions, it is best to have instruction instead of just paddling up and down the pool.

This chart shows ideal weights (in pounds) for males and females. Bone structure influences ideal weight; if a person has a large frame, he or she will weigh more than a person with a small frame, even if they are both the same height. If a person is too heavy or too light and finds it difficult to reduce or gain weight, he or she may have a problem that requires medical attention.

RECOMMENDED WEIGHT FOR FEMALES AND MALES							
FEMALE HEIGHT	SMALL FRAME	MEDIUM FRAME	LARGE FRAME	MALE HEIGHT	SMALL FRAME	MEDIUM FRAME	LARGE FRAME
4'8"	88–94	92–103	100–115	4'8"	101–109	107–111	115–130
4'9"	90–97	94–106	102–118	4'9"	104–112	110–121	118–133
4'10"	92–100	97–109	105–121	4'10"	107–115	113–125	121–136
4'11"	95–103	100–112	109–124	4'11"	110–118	116–128	124–140
5'0"	98–106	103–115	111–127	5'0"	113–121	119–131	127–144
5'1"	101–109	106–118	114–130	5'1"	116–125	122–135	130–148
5'2"	104–112	109–122	117–134	5'2"	120–129	126–139	134–153
5'3"	107–115	112–126	121–138	5'3"	124–133	130–144	139–158
5'4"	110–119	116–131	125–142	5'4"	128–137	134–148	143–162
5'5"	114–123	120–135	129 146	5'5"	132–142	138–152	147–166
5'6"	118–127	124–139	133–150	5'6"	136–146	142–157	151–171
5'7"	122–131	128–143	137–154	5'7"	140–150	146–162	156–176
5'8"	126–136	132–147	141–157	5'8"	144–154	150–167	160–181
5'9"	130–140	136–151	145–164	5'9"	148–158	154–172	165–186
5'10"	134–144	140–155	149–169	5'10"	152–162	159–177	170–191
5'11"	138–148	144–159	153–174	5'11"	156–167	164–182	174–196
6'0"	142–152	149–163	157–179	6'0"	160–171	169–187	178–201

Ice hockey is an exciting sport and good for overall fitness, but protective gear is essential to avoid injury.

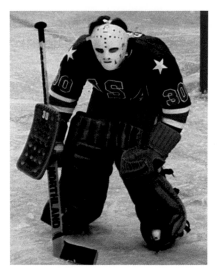

ACTIVITY	AEROBIC BENEFIT	MUSCLE DEVELOPMENT	FLEXIBILITY
EFFECTIVENESS OF SPORTS AND ACTIVITIES FOR PROMOTING FITNESS (ON A SCALE OF 1 TO 10)			
Badminton	7	6	8
Baseball	3	3	4
Basketball	9	7	6
Bicycling	9	8	4
Calisthenics	5	8	10
Football	7	9	5
Golf	4	4	4
Gymnastics	5	9	9
Handball	9	7	8
Hockey (ice)	9	6	5
Horseback riding	6	6	4
Ice skating	9	7	7
Jogging	10	7	4
Judo	7	7	10
Karate	7	8	8
Racquetball	9	7	8
Roller skating	8	6	7
Rowing	10	10	6
Skiing (cross-country)	10	9	7
Skiing (downhill)	8	9	7
Soccer	9	6	5
Softball (slow-pitch)	3	3	4
Squash	9	7	8
Surfing	5	6	6
Swimming	10	7	8
Table tennis	5	5	7
Tennis	8	7	6
Walking	7	6	4
Weight lifting	4	10	4

increase in insulin dosage, or hypoglycemic attacks will be likely to occur. Their blood sugar levels must be carefully monitored.

Other activities that condition the body and are fun to do are dancing, roller skating, ice skating, cycling, hiking, and walking. It is important for an individual to choose an activity that he or she really enjoys and can strive to be better at.

Cross-training

One problem with physical fitness activities is that young people often are bored by a regular routine. This can be overcome by cross-training—adding something challenging and new to an existing sport or activity. Cross-country hiking might make a good outdoor activity, or ice skating a good indoor one.

An individual could also combine walking with jogging, or slow walking with brisk walking. Someone who is a steady runner might enjoy a Swedish routine: instead of jogging at an even pace, one can sprint, skip, jog, or walk to suit one's mood.

Another great aerobic exercise is jumping rope. Steady rope-skipping is of greater aerobic value than jogging. The faster a person skips, the faster the heart will beat. This is a good way of warming up on cold days. To avoid overstraining, a gradual buildup is necessary with this activity.

Many people are attracted to martial arts, such as tai chi, karate, and kung fu (which combine mental and physical disciplines), and to yoga (which makes the body supple and relaxes the mind). These activities add a spiritual dimension to fitness that many people find calming. New exercises and activities help maintain fitness and activity throughout life.

SEE ALSO

AEROBICS • BACKACHE • BLOOD PRESSURE • DIET • EXERCISE • FOOD AND NUTRITION • HEART • ISOMETRIC EXERCISES • JOGGING • JOINT DISORDERS • LETHARGY • MUSCLE • OXYGEN • SPORTS • SPORTS INJURIES • YOGA

Physical Therapy

Physical therapy is the treatment of disease, disability, and injury by physical means, often in conjunction with drugs. It plays an extremely important part in rehabilitation. Physical therapy includes exercise, massage, manipulation, and treatment with water (hydrotherapy), heat, electricity, and ultrasound to restore or maintain mobility and function. Therapists also teach breathing techniques to prevent or alleviate chest infections. Most physical therapists are trained medical personnel who work in hospitals, but some therapists make house calls or work in clinics. Some therapists specialize in sports injuries and work in health clubs or sports clinics; others specialize in the care of handicapped children in special schools.

Manipulation, massage, and mobilization

The techniques used in physical therapy are designed to improve the functioning and increase the strength of various parts of the body. In manipulation, finger and hand movements are used to apply pressure to make joints and tissues more flexible. Manipulation can help realign joints that are slightly out of alignment, for example, and relieve pain where a nerve has become pinched. A great deal of anatomical training is needed to know precisely where and how to apply this pressure.

In massage, the hands manipulate soft tissues around the joints to improve blood flow and help limb movement. Massage relieves muscle pain and helps the patient relax. Mobilization exercises help restore strength to weak muscles.

Hydrotherapy, heat, electricity, and ultrasound

Hydrotherapy involves carrying out exercises in warm pools. The heat of the water helps muscles relax and relieves pain. Paralyzed people particularly benefit from this treatment. The water gives them buoyancy and a greatly increased freedom of movement, while the exercises strengthen their working muscles.

Ultrasound waves passed into the body help reduce inflammation and improve circulation. Infrared radiation, which applies local heat, also improves circulation and at the same time relieves pain. Electric currents reduce pain, improve circulation, and help muscle contractions in diseased and injured limbs.

Q & A

My grandfather recently had a stroke and has lost movement and feeling in his right arm. How can physical therapy help him when he cannot feel anything?

Physical therapists are trained to treat not only loss of movement but also loss of sensation. They will be able to help your grandfather by retraining the nerve pathways that have been affected by the stroke to adapt to new patterns of movement.

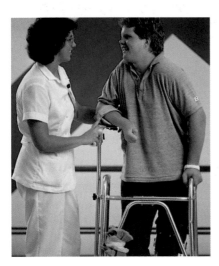

Accustomed to exercise and freedom of movement, athletes are often frustrated by their slow recovery from injuries. Physical therapists have to be good counselors, too.

SEE ALSO

CIRCULATORY SYSTEM • EXERCISE • ISOMETRIC EXERCISES • JOINTS • MASSAGE • MUSCLE • PAIN • SPORTS INJURIES

Podiatry

Podiatry is a practice concerned with all aspects of the care of the feet and with the treatment of commonly occurring minor foot disorders. Podiatrists (formerly called chiropodists) are medically qualified people who specialize in the diagnosis and treatment of diseases and disorders of the feet.

Q & A

I was sick recently and had to spend a lot of time in bed. Now that I'm able to get up, my feet are flat and painful to walk on. Is this permanent?

No. This is a temporary condition. Because you have not been using the muscles in your feet, they have become flabby and weak and cannot support the arches. A podiatrist can give you some foot exercises to strengthen the muscles and help build up the arches.

I am training to be a ballet dancer. I have constant problems with my feet, especially bunions. What can I do to prevent or reduce the effects of strain on my toes?

It is important for you to see a podiatrist regularly, especially if you are planning to have a career in ballet. The podiatrist will check to see that your ballet slippers fit correctly and will advise you on general foot care.

Conditions treated by podiatrists

Corns are protective responses to undue local pressure, usually from unsuitable footwear. The thickening and hardening of the surface layers of the skin lead to a progressive worsening of the condition, because the pressure forces the hard layer deeper into the skin. Simply cutting off or softening a corn will not cure the condition as long as the original cause persists.

In the case of plantar warts (warts on the sole of the foot), the pressure from body weight drives them inward. A podiatrist relieves pressure on the wart while local applications to destroy it are taking effect.

Bunions are also induced by pressure; in this condition, inflammation occurs in the protective, fluid-filled tissue bag (bursa) that lies over the side of the main joint of the big toe. If ill-fitting shoes have forced the tip of the big toe toward the little toe, the sharp angle formed will suffer increased local pressure from the shoe, and the bursa will be inflamed.

Podiatrists can also treat ingrown toenails. This condition is due to pressure or injury that causes the nail to curve under and cut into surrounding tissue. It may also be due to infection that causes inflammation of the tissues at the edge of the nail. These tissues become swollen and overgrow the nail edge.

Onychogryphosis is abnormal thickening of the toenails. It may be due to fungal infection of the nail or to repeated injury. Fungal infection of the nails is common but difficult to cure.

Other conditions commonly treated include flatfoot, athlete's foot, hammertoe, curly toe, clubfoot, ulceration from varicose veins, and gout.

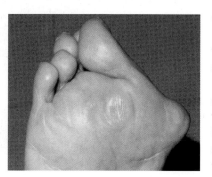

The big toe is turned at an extreme angle, causing deformity of the bone. The soft tissue around it has thickened to form a painful bunion. A podiatrist will carry out surgery to rectify these conditions.

> **SEE ALSO**
>
> **ATHLETE'S FOOT • FEET • JOINTS • MUSCLE • SPORTS INJURIES**

Posture

Posture is the term for the way people stand, sit, and move. In an upright position, the body's center of gravity (where the weight is balanced) is on the lower back and hips. Good posture involves maintaining the balance of body weight around this area, even when people walk, sit, run, work, or play games.

Many people who do not lead active lives have poor posture. Sitting hunched over a desk or at the wheel of a car throws the body weight forward onto the upper spine and shoulders. Many children develop bad posture as they are growing. Boys and girls who are taller than their friends often droop the head and chest and slouch instead of standing up straight.

Achieving good posture

Good posture is not hard to achieve, and a series of simple exercises can help correct bad posture. Dancing, yoga, and body-conditioning systems, such as Pilates or the Alexander technique, can also help. The ideal posture is a straight spine with the back of the shoulders and the back of the buttocks in line. The shoulders should be relaxed and drawn gently back, with the eyes looking straight ahead. It may help to imagine a string coming out of the top of the head and being pulled up; this is the body's natural alignment. It is also best to relax a little to avoid looking stiff. The posture will then improve and people will begin to move more gracefully.

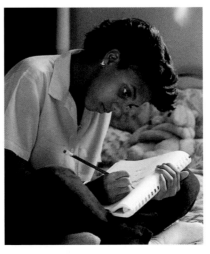

A great benefit of good posture is that it makes people look and feel good. Dancers, models, and actors are aware of this; they look better when they stand and move well. Another benefit is that people with good posture are much less likely to suffer from complaints such as backache and arthritis as they grow older.

This girl may be an excellent student, but sitting hunched over her work will make her feel tired and may cause curvature of the spine. It is always best to sit upright at a desk when studying.

SEE ALSO

ALEXANDER TECHNIQUE • ARTHRITIS • BACKACHE • HIP • JOINT DISORDERS • PHYSICAL FITNESS • SCOLIOSIS • SHOULDER • SKELETAL SYSTEM • SPINAL COLUMN • YOGA

Protein

Protein, contained in foods such as meat, fish, dairy products, and beans, is an important part of the diet. Although protein can be burned in the cells simply as fuel (energy) in the same way as fats and carbohydrates, it has a far more important role. Protein is essential in maintaining the body's continuing process of repairing and rebuilding cells in the body, so that the bones, muscles, and tissues remain in a healthy condition.

Proteins are the body's building blocks and play a vital role in the overall function of the body. Tissues are basically made of protein; the substance that holds together the organs and tissues is a type of protein called collagen; enzymes are made of proteins; and proteins are present both in the blood and in hormones. Proteins are made from amino acids. Different kinds of proteins are combinations of some of the 20 different types of amino acids. The genetic code—which determines everything from a person's hair color to inherited talents—instructs the cells how to combine the amino acids to make proteins. The breakdown and buildup of new protein take place in the body all the time. The entire protein structure of the body is renewed every 60 days. The blood, liver, and other tissues are renewed by food and recycled body proteins.

A high-protein diet is particularly important for babies and children, whose bodies are growing quickly. A baby gets most of its protein from milk. An adult, however, needs less protein.

Q & A

My friend says that she wants to cut out proteins from her diet. What happens if a person doesn't eat any protein?

Protein is an essential part of the diet. If people are starving, they usually do not have enough protein or energy-producing food, so the body breaks down its own protein to act as a fuel, losing much muscle bulk. Lack of protein in a normal-calorie diet leads to a condition called kwashiorkor, which occurs mainly in young children.

Is protein the best sort of food to eat if I want to put on weight and build myself up?

If you want to build up your body's muscle content and strength, the best way is to exercise to encourage the muscles to grow. Simply eating more protein is an expensive way of putting on fat.

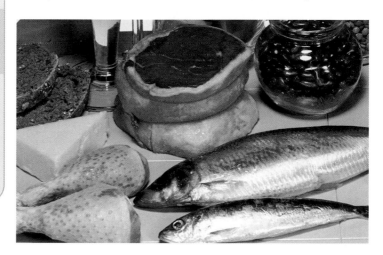

The amount of protein in certain foods can come as a surprise. Dried soybeans, for example, contain more protein weight for weight than a prime cut of beef. Cheese, lentils, and oily fish such as mackerel and herring are also excellent sources of protein.

SEE ALSO

BODY SYSTEMS • CALORIES • CARBOHYDRATES • DIET • DIETING • FATS • FOOD AND NUTRITION • MALNUTRITION • NUTRITIONAL DISEASES • OBESITY

Puberty

Puberty is the name given to the age when children start to become sexually mature. The period from puberty to maturity is called adolescence. During this time, boys and girls go through a number of physical and emotional changes.

Q & A

My brother has hit puberty and now just stays in his room playing music. He hardly talks to anyone in the family at all. Should our parents make him spend time with the rest of the family?

Privacy is very important to some adolescents. It gives them the chance for individual mental development and later emotional balance. Your parents should try to be sympathetic to your brother's needs but make it clear to him that they are there for him and are willing to discuss any worries he might have. You will find that gentle coaxing will be more effective than an argument.

Is chubbiness during puberty caused by malfunctioning glands?

Very rarely. Usually chubbiness is due to a lack of coordination between appetite and need. When children are growing fast, usually between ages 11 and 17, they need more food than before they started puberty. The trouble is that when this growth spurt slows down, the appetite does not always readjust.

Hormonal changes

Puberty is triggered by hormones from the pituitary gland at the base of the brain, which causes changes in the adrenal glands and in the ovaries and testes. In girls, the pituitary gland begins to secrete a variety of stimulating (tropic) hormones, under the influence of another part of the brain called the hypothalamus. These hormones travel to other hormone-secreting (endocrine) glands, which then release other hormones that directly affect sexual development.

Tropic hormones in the ovaries trigger the production of the hormones estrogen and progesterone. In turn, these hormones initiate and maintain the menstrual cycle. Along with the hormones released by the adrenal glands, estrogen and progesterone cause changes in a girl's body shape and stimulate other secondary sexual changes.

As in girls, the pituitary gland is responsible for starting and continuing the changes in a boy's body during puberty. Sperm production is triggered by the action of the tropic hormones on the testes, stimulating the release of the hormone testosterone. Testosterone, along with other hormones from the adrenal glands, causes other secondary sexual developments, such as rapid growth, a deepening voice, and a broadening of the shoulders.

Physical changes

Puberty in a girl may begin as early as age 9 or 10, or be delayed until 15 or even later. Changes in a girl's breasts are an early sign of puberty. Hair begins to grow in the pubic region and in the armpits. As she grows taller, the hips, thighs, and buttocks grow comparatively larger and the waist becomes more defined. The oil-producing glands in her skin become more active, possibly leading to greasy hair and skin.

After some of these changes, a girl will have her first menstrual period. At first, the periods may be slight and come at irregular intervals, but after a year or so, they should settle down to a regular cycle of about 28 days.

Boys usually begin puberty around the age of 13, although it may be as late as 15, with the first ejaculation of semen. During a boy's growth spurt, his legs grow longer, the body's trunk becomes longer and broadens, and the muscles develop. An

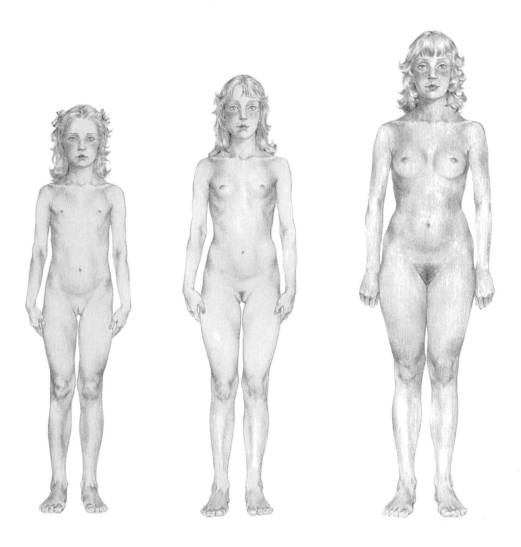

The bodily changes that take place in a girl during puberty can start as early as 9 or 10. The girl shown here has started to develop pubic hair and breasts at the same time. This is not always the case. Often breast development outpaces hair growth in the armpits and pubic region. The illustration charts the progress of a developing girl over a period of about five years.

obvious change is the deepening of the voice. Hair begins to grow in the pubic region and in the armpits, and later on the upper lip and chin. At this time, many boys and girls develop the habit of masturbation. Boys have nocturnal emissions of semen in their sleep, often associated with sexual dreams. Such dreams are normal. Boys, like girls, tend to develop oilier skin and hair and some develop acne due to hormonal changes.

Many girls and boys have mood swings; they are self-conscious and preoccupied with their looks and with their relationships. Some immerse themselves in sports or schoolwork and avoid the opposite sex, who can make them feel unsure of themselves. A great deal of anxiety can be spared if girls and boys know in advance what is happening to them.

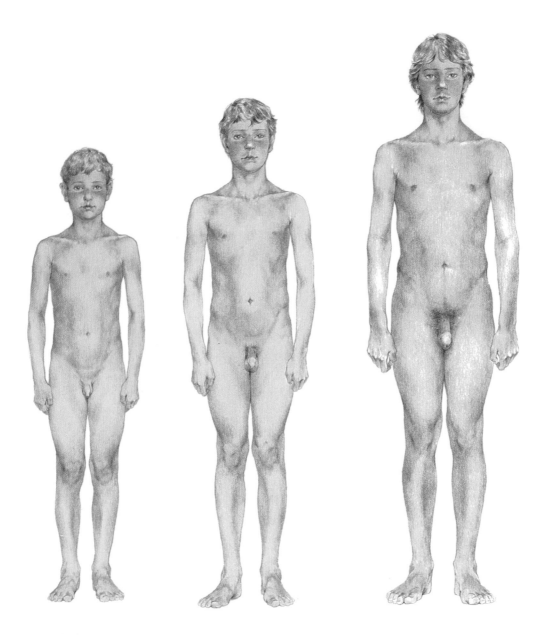

The bodily changes that take place in a boy during puberty can start as early as age 13. Once puberty begins, a boy's body gradually changes shape. The boy also starts genital development and pubic hair growth. This illustration charts the development of a boy from about age 10 to age 16.

SEE ALSO

ANOREXIA AND BULIMIA • BODY SYSTEMS • DIET • DIETING • EXERCISE • FOOD AND NUTRITION • GLANDS • GROWTH • MUSCLE • PHYSICAL EXAMINATION • PHYSICAL FITNESS • POSTURE • SKELETAL SYSTEM • SKIN • SPORTS • WEIGHT CONTROL

Reflexes

When a person touches a stove that is very hot, his or her hand moves away at once. If there is a brilliant flash of light, a person blinks. These are examples of reflex actions. Reflexes are automatic responses of the body to outside influences. They are not under conscious control.

New babies have several reflexes. For example, if someone gently strokes around the mouth of a newborn baby with one finger, the baby will try to suck the finger.

Many reflexes are learned, such as avoiding a hot stove. Some learned reflexes are known as conditioned reflexes. In a conditioned reflex, the desired reaction is brought about by a stimulus that is different from the stimulus that originally caused the reaction.

A Russian psychologist, Ivan Pavlov (1849–1936), was the first person to discover conditioned reflexes. Pavlov found that if he rang a bell every time he gave a dog a scrap of food, after a while the dog would salivate if Pavlov merely rang the bell without any food being in sight.

Q & A

Do young babies have a sucking reflex or do they learn to suck?

Babies are born with a sucking reflex. If you gently stroke the cheek of a newborn baby near the mouth, his or her head will turn toward your finger. Once the finger is in his or her mouth, the sucking reflex is stimulated. The reflex is lost as the child grows.

I find myself blinking a lot when I walk into a strong light. Is the blinking a reflex?

Yes. Strong light will cause a reflex blink, giving the pupil a chance to constrict (again by reflex). Blinking avoids overstimulation of the retina, which might otherwise be damaged by excessive light.

My friend says that it's possible to stop reflexes from occurring. Is she right?

Yes and no. For example, simple tendon reflexes can be inhibited by tensing the muscles. Others, such as the choking reflex, cannot be stopped at will.

By striking just below the knee with a tendon hammer (right), the doctor can test muscle reflexes.

Blinking (below) is a reflex action that protects the retina from strong light.

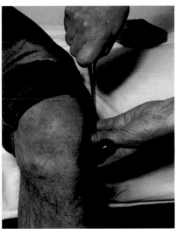

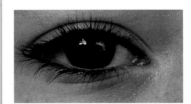

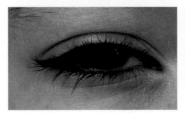

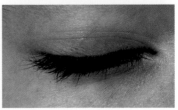

SEE ALSO

KNEE • MUSCLE • NERVOUS SYSTEM • PAIN • TENDON

Respiratory System

Q & A

My brother has been diagnosed as having small lungs. Is this serious?

Each lung has a capacity of around 0.09 cubic foot (2.5 l), but the amount of air passing in and out is often only a tenth of this, so your brother should be all right. Many people manage with only one lung.

Why are singers taught to breathe from the diaphragm?

The diaphragm controls breathing rate and depth. A voice teacher helps students develop their abdominal muscles to control their diaphragm so that they can hold long notes and create vibrato.

I broke my ribs playing basketball. Why was I not bandaged or given any treatment?

Although broken or cracked ribs can be uncomfortable or painful, the main danger is that the chest movement will be reduced, producing less airflow into and out of the underlying lung. This can cause pneumonia, so it is unusual to bandage broken ribs.

All body cells need a constant supply of oxygen to survive and to dispose of a waste product, carbon dioxide. Both requirements are fulfilled by the respiratory system and the circulatory system. The two systems deliver oxygen from the lungs to the cells and remove carbon dioxide from the cells for return to the lungs, where it is exhaled. This exchange of oxygen and carbon dioxide between the air, blood, and tissues of the body is known as respiration.

When air is breathed in, it is taken to the lungs. There, the oxygen it contains is exchanged for carbon dioxide, which, with water vapor, is expelled when people breathe out. This process is controlled by nerves that automatically send impulses to the muscles, so that people breathe in and out in an involuntary way.

Air is drawn into the body through the nose and mouth and travels down the throat (the pharynx and larynx) and the windpipe (trachea). The windpipe divides into two branches called bronchi, each leading to a lung.

How the respiratory system works

The lungs are like a pair of bellows in the chest. Around them are the rib cage and the rib muscles. Below them is a sheet of muscle called the diaphragm. The rib cage, muscles, and diaphragm form the chest cavity. When the diaphragm contracts and the chest wall rises, the space in the chest increases and air rushes into the lungs. When the muscles relax, the lungs, which are naturally elastic, collapse and air rushes out.

From the nostrils to the lungs, the air is warmed, moistened, and filtered. Tiny hairs covered with mucus line the passages and trap as much dust and germs as possible when they enter the system. However, these hairs cannot cope with cigarette smoke or very polluted air. If a large particle enters the system, it is coughed out or sneezed out. Food is prevented from entering the respiratory system by the epiglottis, a flap of tissue that closes off the windpipe as the food passes into the gullet.

The air travels into the bronchi and then into even smaller branches called bronchioles. At the ends of these narrow tubes are minute air sacs called alveoli. The alveoli are covered with a network of tiny blood vessels called capillaries. The exchange of gases—oxygen for carbon dioxide—takes place through the walls of the alveoli, which are fused with the capillary walls.

The red blood cells contain hemoglobin, a compound that picks up the oxygen from the lungs. The hemoglobin carries the oxygen to every cell in the body and releases it. At the same time, carbon dioxide passes into the blood and is carried back to the lungs, where it is breathed out.

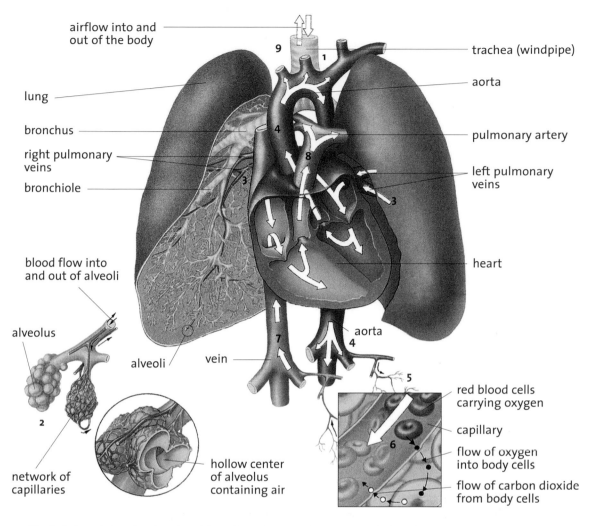

airflow into and out of the body

trachea (windpipe)

aorta

lung

bronchus

pulmonary artery

right pulmonary veins

left pulmonary veins

bronchiole

blood flow into and out of alveoli

heart

alveolus

aorta

alveoli

vein

red blood cells carrying oxygen

capillary

flow of oxygen into body cells

network of capillaries

hollow center of alveolus containing air

flow of carbon dioxide from body cells

Air (1) inhaled via the trachea (windpipe), bronchi, and bronchioles reaches the alveoli, where oxygen from the air is transferred to the capillaries surrounding each alveolus (2). The oxygenated blood is carried by the pulmonary veins (3) to the left side of the heart and pushed into the aorta (4), which is the body's main artery. Blood then travels around the body through the arteries to the capillaries (5). The oxygen carried by the red blood cells is given to the body cells, which transfer their waste product, carbon dioxide, to the fluid of the blood (6). This blood is carried back through the veins (7) into the right side of the heart. Finally, the blood flows through the pulmonary artery (8) into the lungs. At the site of the alveoli (2), the circulating blood gives up its carbon dioxide, which is exhaled (9), and then takes in oxygen again (1). The cycle then repeats itself.

SEE ALSO

ASTHMA • AUTONOMIC NERVOUS SYSTEM • BODY SYSTEMS • CIRCULATORY SYSTEM • HEART • HYPERVENTILATION • MUSCLE • NERVOUS SYSTEM • OXYGEN

Rest and Relaxation

Rest and relaxation are ways of recharging the body's batteries and guarding against stress. Knowing how to relax by getting rid of mental and physical tension is essential to good health. To stay healthy, a person needs to relax mentally and physically. It is difficult for people to achieve their goals if they are so tense that they suffer from stress, or so tired that they cannot move away from the television.

The best way to relax is to be active. The more exercise one gets, the less tired one will feel. The body will also be in good shape, and any emotional and psychological problems that may have been present will become less intense. Jogging and swimming are especially good for lifting a person's mood. If people feel tired or exhausted, they should not head for the refrigerator for a sandwich; instead, they should go to the gym or do some other type of exercise.

Importance of sleep

Being tired from intense physical activity helps people get proper rest when they need it. Young people particularly find it difficult to get out of bed in the morning. Seven or eight hours' sleep is all that is needed. If people go to bed at a reasonable time, they should wake rested and refreshed in the morning. Staying up late—studying or partying—means that people are still tired when they wake and will be unable to concentrate or enjoy the next day's activities.

Avoiding tension by learning to relax

Everyone has to cope with some tension in life. At school, work, or home people constantly experience fear, anger, guilt, overwork, and worry. Some of this tension is necessary if people are to meet

Q & A

How can I relax and still remain alert while driving?

If you have had an exhausting day, pause a few minutes in the driver's seat before you turn on the ignition. Relax all your muscles in turn, and make sure your back is well supported. Lean back when you are driving; do not hunch over the wheel. At stoplights or when you are in dense traffic, check again that your muscles are relaxed.

How can I be, and appear, more relaxed during an interview for an after-school job?

Tension is unavoidable during an interview, and one of the aspects of the interview is for the employer to see how you perform in a tense situation. To appear at ease, sit with your back against the back of the chair, relaxing your shoulders. Keep your feet still and your hands folded in your lap. Do not fold your arms across your chest or lean too far back in your chair.

Regular exercise keeps people in good physical condition and has the added advantage of giving them time to relax and escape from worries.

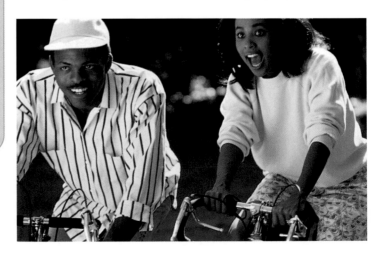

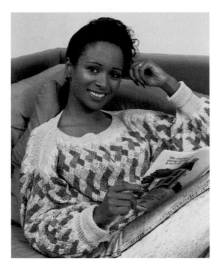

Many people find that one of the best ways to unwind is to relax in a quiet, comfortable room at home. Even a rest of only 15 to 20 minutes helps relieve tension.

Sometimes it is enjoyable doing nothing. It can be restful and relaxing and can make a positive contribution to good health. However, such relaxation should also be balanced by activity.

challenges and achieve ambitions. However, if too much tension builds up, without periods of relaxation, there is a danger of mental illness or the development of a physical problem.

The body's response to relaxation

When people are properly relaxed, a number of changes take place in the body. The heartbeat decreases and breathing becomes slower. The brain-wave patterns are changed and people become more aware of their body and thoughts.

If people suffer from tension, for example before an exam or an interview for a job, they should make a conscious effort to relax the muscles one by one and to clear the mind of conflicting thoughts. Books about relaxation can be found in local libraries or bookstores.

Relieving mental stress

People who suffer from fear, phobias, depression, and other mental problems often benefit from special relaxation programs. They learn simple relaxation techniques, such as deep breathing and how to reduce muscle tension gradually.

Some people find that yoga, meditation, or massage are effective activities in reducing fears and worries, and afterward they feel rested and revitalized.

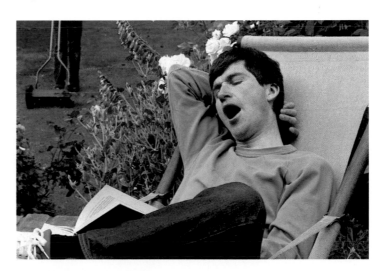

SEE ALSO

EXERCISE • ISOMETRIC EXERCISES • JOGGING • LETHARGY • MASSAGE • PHYSICAL FITNESS • SPORTS • TIREDNESS • YOGA

Salmonella

Salmonellosis is a common form of food poisoning, caused by bacteria of the genus *Salmonella*. These organisms contaminate foods from domestic animals, especially eggs, poultry, meats, and dairy products, as well as fish and shellfish. Salmonella is considered one of the nation's most important communicable diseases, affecting approximately two million people each year.

Q & A

I read somewhere that the acid in a person's stomach destroys salmonella. If this is true, then how do people manage to get infected with salmonella?

It is certainly true that stomach acid provides an important barrier to infection. Food tends to stay in the stomach longer than liquids, so an infected drink may be a greater hazard than infected food. It also appears that people with no stomach acid (as a result of either illness or an operation) are more at risk of being infected by salmonella.

Bacteria killed by heat

Salmonella bacteria are killed by heat. Freshly cooked food that has been heated through quite thoroughly should be safe. However, unless the cook is hygienic, the food may be contaminated again by coming into contact with raw meat, kitchen utensils, or hands. Cooked and raw food should always be kept separate. Freezing does not kill salmonella; it simply stops bacterial growth, which will begin again as the food thaws. Frozen poultry is easily contaminated as it is prepared for freezing; it must always be thawed out completely before cooking, and then cooked thoroughly all the way through. Undercooked eggs, or foods such as mayonnaise that are made with raw eggs, may also carry the infection. These types of foods should not be given to those who are in at-risk groups, such as pregnant women, babies, young children, people with immune deficiency diseases, and seniors.

Some household pets, such as chicks, frogs, and aquarium snails, can pass on salmonella bacteria. Infection can be avoided by careful hygiene. The hands should always be washed after handling aquarium pets, and pet birds should be kept out of the kitchen or other rooms where food is usually prepared or eaten.

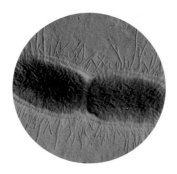

Cooked meat can be contaminated with bacilli from raw meat. The salmonella bacterium seems to thrive in poultry and eggs and in processed cooked meats prepared in unhygienic conditions.

Symptoms and treatments

Symptoms of salmonella poisoning include severe headache, vomiting, diarrhea, stomach cramps, and sometimes fever. Treatment is usually bed rest with a diet of bland food and plenty of fluids. Patients at risk are often prescribed antibiotics.

Epidemics of salmonella poisoning can be particularly dangerous in nursing homes, where the elderly patients are vulnerable to it. Public health regulations aim to prevent outbreaks by overseeing standards of hygiene in food preparation factories, hospitals, restaurants, and hotels.

SEE ALSO

DIGESTIVE SYSTEM DISEASES AND DISORDERS • FOOD POISONING

Salt

Salt is essential to life. It plays a part in stabilizing the body's acid and alkaline balance; helps in the maintenance of muscles, nerves, and blood; and, with potassium, regulates the body's internal fluid supply. Salt is a compound of sodium and chlorine and is naturally present in most of the foods eaten. However, in the United States and elsewhere in the developed world, people have become accustomed to well-salted food. Salt is also added to meat and vegetables in the cooking process. There are extremely high levels of salt in foods such as processed potato chips, peanuts, snacks, and other junk foods. Surprisingly large amounts of salt are hidden in breads, cereals, and canned foods.

Nutritionists agree that people eat too much salt and that this could be the cause of a number of conditions, such as fluid retention, kidney disorders, and even muscle damage. Many of the symptoms of premenstrual syndrome are in part due to the retention of salt and water in the body. Salt has also been linked with migraine headaches. Excessive salt can cause hypertension (high blood pressure) in some people, which may lead in turn to heart diseases and strokes. Populations that eat low-salt diets have a much reduced incidence of hypertension.

People should cut down or give up salt to minimize the risks of disease in later life. In cooking, it is best to season food only with spices, herbs, garlic, and lemon juice to add flavor.

Q & A

Is it true that too much salt causes high blood pressure?

The exact cause of high blood pressure is not known, but it is likely to be due to a few factors, including heredity. There is also some evidence to suggest that salt may be an important factor. For example, the disease is more common in countries where there is a high salt intake. There is little doubt that the body's salt-retaining mechanisms are involved in setting the level of blood pressure higher than normal. Very low-salt diets can also be successful in lowering blood pressure.

I often get cramps in my legs at night. Could this be caused by a lack of salt?

Probably not. Severe salt loss can bring about cramps, but this is unlikely in a temperate climate. Night cramps are common and can be alleviated by taking quinine pills before going to bed.

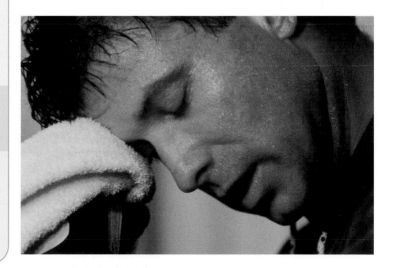

Athletes need more salt in their diets, because they lose a great deal of salt and fluid through sweating, both of which need to be replaced to avoid dehydration.

SEE ALSO

DIET • FOOD AND NUTRITION • MINERALS • MUSCLE DISEASES AND DISORDERS • NUTRITIONAL DISEASES • STROKE

Sciatica

Q & A

I'm very confused. What is the difference between a backache and sciatica?

Sciatica is the name given to the type of back pain that radiates down the back of the leg. However, herniated (slipped) disks may start with pain limited to the back before the disk starts exerting pressure on the nerves to the leg, which causes sciatica. Most people with a bad back do not have slipped disks; they have strained ligaments and muscles.

I've heard of some people who had surgery to cure their sciatica, but that sounds extreme to me. Is surgery always necessary, or are there other ways to cure sciatica?

For a person's first attack of sciatica, the doctor will probably not recommend surgery so long as he or she is fairly confident that a slipped disk is the cause (as it usually is). Most people with sciatica find that the pain improves if they can rest their back properly and then resume exercise.

Sciatica, or sciatic neuritis, is pain along the large sciatic nerve that runs from the lower back down through the buttocks and along the back of each leg. It is a relatively common form of back pain. The pain is caused by pressure on the sciatic nerve as it leaves the spinal column. Sciatica can have a variety of causes, including a herniated (slipped) disk in the spinal column, arthritis, or a fall. In most people who have sciatica, the disks in the backbone have become weakened, either with age or as a result of excessive strain. The disks are pads of tissue that separate the vertebrae. The disks and vertebrae provide the necessary flexibility for people to stretch and bend. Each disk consists of a soft center, which acts as a shock absorber, and a tough fibrous outer layer. Sometimes, this outer layer weakens in parts, and the soft center bulges out. The resulting bulge puts pressure on the nerve to the leg and causes the pain of sciatica.

Any pressure on the sciatic nerve causes sharp, stabbing pains in the buttock and down the leg. It may happen suddenly when someone is bending or stretching or it may come on gradually. Even a slight movement, such as coughing or sneezing, can bring on the pain or make it worse. For anyone suffering from sciatica, walking and sitting can be painful and difficult. The most comfortable position is lying on the back with the knees bent.

Treatments

Sciatica as a result of a slipped disk, which can be extremely unpleasant on some occasions and often disabling, usually improves on its own if the proper measures are taken. Treatment for sciatica starts with relieving the pain by resting in a firm bed and taking painkillers when necessary. Manual treatments, such as physical therapy and osteopathic or chiropractic treatments, may help relieve the pressure. Painkillers such as nonsteroidal anti-inflammatory drugs (NSAIDs), oral steroids, or epidural steroid injections can help relieve the inflammation. Muscle relaxants may be used to help relieve spasms.

It is very important to stay in bed and to resist the temptation to be up and about when the disk is only half-healed; otherwise, the patient will be back to where he or she started. Surgical treatment, a last resort, is usually reserved for those who have had repeated episodes that have not improved with bed rest.

SEE ALSO

CHIROPRACTIC • LEG • NERVOUS SYSTEM • PAIN • PHYSICAL THERAPY • SLIPPED DISK • SPINAL COLUMN • SPINAL CORD

Scoliosis

Q & A

My 10-year-old-brother has scoliosis. The doctor says that my brother may need an operation when he is older but must wear a brace until then. Why?

Scoliosis tends to worsen during growth, so your brother probably needs a brace to prevent his curve from getting any worse. Operations for scoliosis stop the spine from growing, so surgeons prefer to put off the operation until the child's growth is nearly complete.

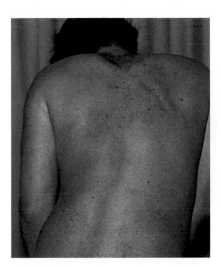

The effects of scoliosis—a twisted spine—can be clearly seen in this woman.

Any sideways curvature seen or felt in the spine (spinal column) is called scoliosis. However, the spine is very flexible, especially in childhood, and it is easily bent to one side. A normal spine should appear straight when viewed from the back. There are other forms of spinal curvature, including kyphosis (a rounded back) and hunched shoulders in people who have poor posture.

There are two types of scoliosis, postural and structural. Postural scoliosis happens when something other than the spine causes it to bend to one side: for example, having one leg shorter than the other. When a child is sitting, however, the spine is straight. This test distinguishes postural scoliosis from the structural form. Many children have slight postural scoliosis without being aware of it. Older people with a slipped disk may have tight muscles on one side of the spine, which can also cause temporary postural scoliosis.

In structural scoliosis, there is a permanent defect in the bones of the spine or in their relationship to each other. In addition, because there is a fixed abnormal curve, there will always be a secondary curve to compensate so that the shoulders remain straight. The most common type of structural scoliosis is adolescent idiopathic scoliosis, which occurs while the spine is growing. The cause is unknown. It is usually first noticed between the ages of 10 and 15 and may affect any part of the spine. If the scoliosis is in the chest region of the spine, the ribs will protrude on the side of the curve and cause a hump. In girls, the breasts may also appear unbalanced.

Other types of structural scoliosis may be due to bone disease, bone abnormalities present from birth, or unbalanced muscle disorders that cause a sideways pull on the spine.

Treatments

First, the type of scoliosis must be diagnosed. X-rays are taken of the spine to measure the angle between the upper surface of vertebrae above and below the scoliosis. Regular checks are needed to monitor the condition. Exercises may be helpful for maintaining the flexibility of the spine, but they cannot cure scoliosis. If the curvature gets worse and the angle exceeds 20 degrees, a spinal support is required until the bones have stopped growing. When the curvature is more than 40 degrees, surgery is required to straighten the spine and fuse the bones.

SEE ALSO

ARTHRITIS • BACKACHE • EXERCISE • GROWTH • POSTURE • SLIPPED DISK • SPINAL COLUMN • SPORTS

Scurvy

Q & A

Is scurvy an extremely painful condition?

If the teeth are still present in the mouth, it can be very painful. The pain of scurvy is most striking in babies. The disease causes bleeding into the periosteum, the fibrous covering of the bones, and this condition is so painful that the baby may adopt the characteristic froglike posture associated with scurvy.

I understand that scurvy causes the teeth to fall out, but what happens if a person has already lost all of his or her teeth?

One of the main effects of scurvy is on the teeth and gums, which bleed and become infected. If the person has already lost his or her teeth, the gums will not be affected.

Is there vitamin C in potatoes?

Yes, but the amount varies according to how long they have been stored. New potatoes contain more vitamin C than older potatoes. Also, prolonged cooking destroys the vitamin.

Scurvy is a disease caused by severe vitamin C deficiency. This vitamin is present mainly in fresh fruits and vegetables. In developed countries, scurvy is uncommon, but elderly people, alcoholics, and anyone who does not eat properly may develop it.

Vitamin C is needed to produce collagen, which is the basic protein that makes up all fibrous tissues in the body. Vitamin C is essential for the formation of blood vessels, bones, teeth, and ligaments. If there is insufficient vitamin C in the diet, blood vessels weaken and may bleed and other collagen problems may arise. Vitamin C is also an important antioxidant, a substance that helps reduce the risk of tissue damage from powerful chemical groups called free radicals. Free radicals are implicated in many disease processes and other health hazards, such as smoking, and are thought to be involved in the deposition of cholesterol in the arteries.

Children who do not have enough vitamin C lose weight and become irritable, their gums bleed, and their limbs may swell and become painful. Adults with scurvy also lose weight and become depressed. Their gums bleed and then draw back from the teeth, which may fall out. Large bruises appear, usually on the thighs, and sometimes there are little red bleeding marks around the roots of body hairs. As the disease gets worse, there is bleeding in the muscles or in the intestines. Wounds may not heal, because vitamin C is essential if the skin is to heal properly. The bones may become softened due to the deficiency.

Treatment for scurvy is simple—vitamin C tablets bring immediate improvement; then the patient must keep to a diet that contains enough vitamin C.

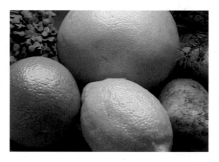

Scurvy was once a common disease among sailors who went on long ocean voyages. However, once it was recognized that eating fresh fruits and vegetables could prevent scurvy, such supplies were carried on board whenever possible.

SEE ALSO

AGING • ANTIOXIDANTS • BRUISES • CHOLESTEROL • CIRCULATORY SYSTEM • DIET • DIGESTIVE SYSTEM • FOOD AND NUTRITION • LIGAMENTS • MUSCLE • NUTRITIONAL DISEASES • PROTEIN • SKIN • VITAMINS

Shoulder

A shoulder is a joint that connects the arm to the body. A ball-shaped projection at the top of the humerus (upper arm bone) rests in a rather shallow cup in the scapula (shoulder blade). This ball-and-socket joint allows the arm to rotate through a complete circle in several planes. No other joint in the body has this range of movement.

The ligaments that hold the shoulder joint in place are not particularly strong, and that is why people often dislocate their shoulders. However, the muscles that control the shoulder's movement help make the shoulder joint stable. The most important muscles are the series of fan-shaped muscles that run from the scapula to the top of the humerus and to the end of the clavicle (collarbone).

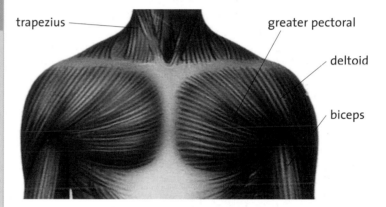

trapezius — greater pectoral — deltoid — biceps

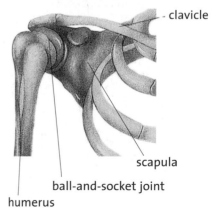

clavicle — scapula — ball-and-socket joint — humerus

The shoulder is a ball and-socket joint. The head of the upper arm bone, or humerus, sits in the shallow socket of the scapula, or shoulder blade. A special fluid contained in the synovial capsule protects and lubricates the joint. The ligaments and muscles hold the humerus and scapula in position.

SEE ALSO

EXERCISE • JOINT DISORDERS • JOINT REPLACEMENT • JOINTS • LIGAMENTS • MUSCLE • SKELETAL SYSTEM • SPORTS INJURIES • TENDON • TENNIS ELBOW

Skeletal System

Q & A

How much force is needed to break a bone?

That varies according to the position, shape, and health of the bone. The long thin bones of the arms and legs are more prone to snapping fractures than are the plate bones of the shoulder and pelvis (which are more prone to heavy blows or crushing injuries). People who are undernourished, and older people whose bones have lost part of their protein framework, have brittle bones that break easily. This is particularly the case with menopausal women who have osteoporisis.

What is a greenstick fracture?

Instead of the bone breaking into two or more separate fragments, only one side of it breaks. The other side is more bent than broken. The appearance and effect are similar to what happens if you try to break a stick of wood that is still green, hence the name. These fractures usually occur only in children whose bones have not yet fully ossified and are thus more supple.

The human skeleton is strong enough to keep the body upright and protect vital organs, yet it is flexible enough to allow great freedom of movement. The skeletal system consists of the skeleton itself, which is made of bones, and the related cartilage, ligaments, and muscles.

An adult's skeleton has 206 bones. As a child grows, many bones—for example, those in the skull—fuse together. Male and female skeletons have the same number of bones, but in general the female skeleton is smaller and lighter. A woman's pelvis is broader and more boat-shaped, giving the hips their characteristic shape and allowing room for the passage of a baby's head during childbirth. A woman's shoulders are relatively narrow. In a man, the general proportions are reversed: broad shoulders and slim hips.

Each part of the skeleton has a different function. The skull protects the brain, the middle ear, the inner ear, and the eyes. The spinal column (backbone) protects the spinal cord and is made up of a chain of small bones, rather like spools, called vertebrae. Its structure gives the spinal column enormous strength, but at the same time it is very flexible. The rib cage, made up of the backbone, sternum (breastbone), and ribs, protects the heart and lungs. The pelvis shields the reproductive organs and the bladder and serves as an anchor point for the legs.

Cartilage

Cartilage is a smooth, tough, flexible tissue that forms part of the skeletal system. It is composed of cells surrounded by fibers of collagen and elastic. Cartilage gives the body strength and elasticity. There are no blood vessels or nerves in cartilage. Instead, food and oxygen are diffused from the surrounding tissue fluid.

The structure of cartilage varies according to its function. Yellow, or elastic, cartilage is extremely flexible and occurs in the earlobes, tip of the nose, and voice-producing part of the larynx. Fibrous cartilage forms the shock absorbers in the knees and the disks between the vertebrae in the spine. Hyaline cartilage lines the movable joints of the body.

Ossification

Nearly all bones begin as rods of cartilage that are gradually hardened by deposits of calcium and other minerals. This process of hardening is called ossification. It begins in the third or fourth month of an embryo's life and continues until about the age of 21. With age and wear and tear, cartilage can cause problems, particularly in the spine and knees.

Skeletal development

A newborn baby has more bones in its body than an adult. At birth, a baby has about 350 bones; over the years, some of these bones fuse into larger units. A baby's skull is a good example of this. During birth, the skull is squeezed through a narrow canal. If the skull were as inflexible as an adult's, it would be impossible for the baby to pass through the mother's pelvic outlet. The fontanelles, or gaps between the sections of the skull, allow the skull to be molded sufficiently to fit the birth canal. After birth, the baby's fontanelles gradually close.

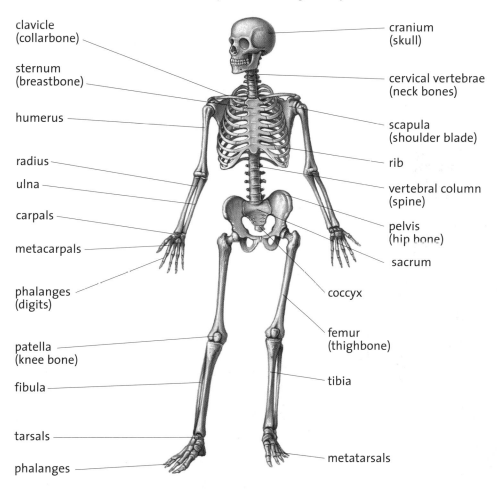

clavicle (collarbone)

sternum (breastbone)

humerus

radius

ulna

carpals

metacarpals

phalanges (digits)

patella (knee bone)

fibula

tarsals

phalanges

cranium (skull)

cervical vertebrae (neck bones)

scapula (shoulder blade)

rib

vertebral column (spine)

pelvis (hip bone)

sacrum

coccyx

femur (thighbone)

tibia

metatarsals

The human skeleton, made up of more than 200 rigid but living bones, supports the body and its vital organs and provides its shape. Here, the major bones of the skeleton are identified.

SEE ALSO

ELBOW • FEET • HIP • JOINTS • KNEE • LEG • LIGAMENTS • MUSCLE • SHOULDER • SPINAL COLUMN • TENDON

Skin

The skin is an organ—the largest the body has. It not only protects the body from injury and infection but also keeps the body's temperature and moisture content stable. Through its network of sensory nerve endings, the skin picks up information about external stimuli for transmission to the brain. The skin enables people to feel things and to experience painful and pleasant sensations through touch.

The skin is also a good indicator of the body's general health, because it is affected from within by the food eaten, by stress levels, by hormonal balance, and by physical illness. A clear, glowing complexion is regarded as a sign of good health, whereas a pallid skin could suggest anemia and a yellow tone could indicate jaundice.

Structure of the skin
The skin consists of two parts: the epidermis and the dermis. The epidermis is the upper (outer) part of the skin. It has several layers of cells, which are formed in the lower part, the dermis. Skin cells are constantly moving up to the surface, where they die and are formed into a material called keratin, which is finally shed as tiny, barely visible scales. The dermis contains the sweat glands, sebaceous glands, apocrine glands, hair follicles, and nerves. The hairs and ducts from the glands pass through the epidermis to the surface. The apocrine glands are present in the armpits and other places and produce an odor.

Skin is categorized as oily, dry, or normal, but some people have combination skin, with both oily and dry patches, usually on the face. Oily skin is more prone to problems such as acne during adolescence and early adulthood, but it ages better than dry skin, which wrinkles easily.

Skin color is due to the pigment melanin, which is produced in the lowest layer of the epidermis. The pigment-producing cells are larger in dark-skinned people than in fair-skinned people, but the number of these cells is the same. However, the amount of melanin produced varies, with dark-skinned people producing more melanin than fair-skinned people. The pigment-producing cells are also responsible for freckles.

Moles
Moles are dark spots made of collections of pigmented cells. They are very common and can be found anywhere on the body. Moles may be large or small, raised or flat, smooth or scaly, hairy or hairless. Most moles are present at birth or develop slowly during childhood. They may grow larger or darker in late adolescence or when a woman is pregnant.

Q & A

What factors affect how fast skin ages?

Inheritance is probably the most important factor in skin aging. Other influences involved are the environment, such as the amount of sun damage, and hormonal changes throughout life. The loss of elasticity that causes wrinkles in old age is due to changes in the fibers of the supporting layer of skin. Skin also becomes drier and hair becomes thinner with age.

SHAVING

During puberty, which starts at any time from age 13 to age 15, boys begin to develop facial hair. The amount of hair that grows depends on coloring and hormones. Blond men often have only a slight growth of hair, whereas those with darker hair often have a thick, dense growth. Most men prefer to remove facial hair by daily shaving.

Women often shave the hair under their arms, and those who have noticeable hair on their legs may shave them as well. To remove unwanted hair on other parts of the body, other methods of hair removal are often more suitable.

Most moles are harmless, but if a mole changes at all after adolescence, particularly if it bleeds or itches, it must be shown to a doctor. New moles that appear on adults should also be examined by a doctor. Sometimes, they may develop into a kind of skin cancer—malignant melanoma—and must be removed by surgery as soon as possible to prevent them from spreading.

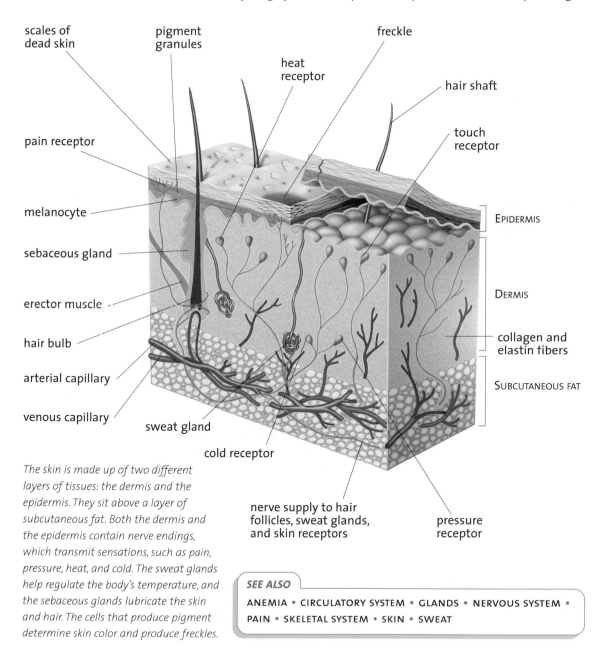

scales of dead skin

pigment granules

freckle

heat receptor

hair shaft

pain receptor

touch receptor

melanocyte

EPIDERMIS

sebaceous gland

DERMIS

erector muscle

collagen and elastin fibers

hair bulb

SUBCUTANEOUS FAT

arterial capillary

venous capillary

sweat gland

cold receptor

nerve supply to hair follicles, sweat glands, and skin receptors

pressure receptor

The skin is made up of two different layers of tissues: the dermis and the epidermis. They sit above a layer of subcutaneous fat. Both the dermis and the epidermis contain nerve endings, which transmit sensations, such as pain, pressure, heat, and cold. The sweat glands help regulate the body's temperature, and the sebaceous glands lubricate the skin and hair. The cells that produce pigment determine skin color and produce freckles.

SEE ALSO

ANEMIA • CIRCULATORY SYSTEM • GLANDS • NERVOUS SYSTEM • PAIN • SKELETAL SYSTEM • SKIN • SWEAT

Slipped Disk

Between two vertebrae of the spinal column is a disk of jellylike material, surrounded by a tough outer layer. The disk connects the vertebrae and acts as a cushion between them. Sometimes everyday wear and tear or a sudden strain makes the tough outer layer crack open. The inner layer bulges out and may press on a nerve as it leaves the spinal cord. This condition is known as a slipped or prolapsed disk. It can cause severe backache. In some cases, any movement is very painful; even coughing or sneezing can cause a sharp pain. The muscles along the spine may go into spasm or become weak or even paralyzed. The symptoms may appear suddenly or they may build up over several weeks.

The most commonly affected disks are in the lower part of the back, where the greatest strains occur, but disks in any part of the back or neck can crack open.

Most people recover from a slipped disk simply by lying flat in bed. The soft inner disk material tends to dry and shrink once it has prolapsed, thus relieving the pressure on the nerve. Lying flat keeps the pressure within the disk to a minimum. In a standing position, this pressure is higher. It is best to put a board under a soft mattress—or even put the mattress on the floor—to prevent the back from bending. In severe cases, patients may need bed rest and pain relief for two weeks or more. Great patience is needed; getting up too soon often results in a relapse.

If the patient is free of pain, physical therapy can help. If the disk is in the neck, the patient may need to wear a collar support. Painkillers and muscle relaxants will ease the pain.

In a few cases, the damaged disk may have to be removed by surgery. Patients are usually mobile again after about two weeks.

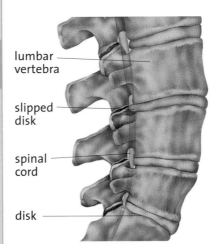

lumbar vertebra

slipped disk

spinal cord

disk

A slipped disk occurs when the soft inner core of a spinal disk bulges out and presses on a nerve, causing muscle weakness and pain.

SEE ALSO

BACKACHE • MUSCLE • PAIN • PHYSICAL THERAPY • SCIATICA • SPINAL COLUMN • SPINAL CORD

Q & A

Does sleeping with a board under the mattress help prevent a slipped disk?

No, sleeping with a board under the mattress will not prevent a slipped disk. However, many people with back problems find that a firm mattress helps their back, because it is more comfortable. A soft mattress can sag in the middle, so that lying on the bed bends the back. This is an uncomfortable position. Putting a hard board under a soft mattress is an inexpensive and effective way to increase comfort.

Are women more prone to slipped disks than men?

No. Two to three times as many men as women suffer from a slipped disk. The reasons for this are not clear, and contrary to popular belief, heavy physical work is not associated with a greater risk of a slipped disk. However, a slipped disk is obviously more troublesome to someone who does heavy manual work than to someone with a more sedentary lifestyle, such as an office worker.

Spinal Column

The spinal column, or backbone, is the main bony support of the body. At the top, the spinal column supports the head. At the lower end, it is linked to the pelvis.

The spine consists of 33 small bones called vertebrae, which are stacked on top of each other to form the spinal column. The vertebrae are separated by disks with an outer fibrous ring and an inner pulpy center. These pulpy centers act as cushions and allow the spine to bend slightly. The spinal canal is a continuous channel that holds and protects the nerves that form the spinal cord. The spinal cord is further protected by membranes and is surrounded by a liquid called cerebrospinal fluid, which acts as a shock absorber.

Of the 33 bones, 24 are movable. Seven bones form the neck and are known as the cervical vertebrae. Below them are 12 thoracic (chest) vertebrae and five lumbar (lower back) vertebrae. At the lower end are two groups of bones that are fused together to form two bones (the sacrum and the coccyx).

Spinal injuries

The most common spinal injuries are a slipped disk (in which the pulpy content of the cartilage cushions moves out of place) and a fracture of the spine. A slipped disk is painful, but a fracture of the spine may cause injury to the spinal cord and lead to paralysis. A patient with a suspected fracture of the spine must be moved very carefully to avoid damaging the nerves.

Q & A

Is the spinal column always damaged by a broken neck?

Not always. However, spinal column damage often does occur when a person's neck is broken. The spinal cord can also be injured without there ever being a fracture of the spinal bones. This situation tends to happen when the cord is suddenly stretched or twisted in an accident. More important than the fracture is whether any bones are displaced, causing them to press onto the cord in the spinal canal that runs through the spinal bones.

My grandmother, who is 63, recently told me that she is shrinking. She says she is 2 inches (5 cm) shorter now than she was 40 years ago. I believe her, but how can she possibly be shrinking?

As the body ages, the bones in the vertebral column get smaller and the disks of cartilage between them get thinner and harder. This makes the disks shrink in size; with bone shrinkage, the person becomes shorter.

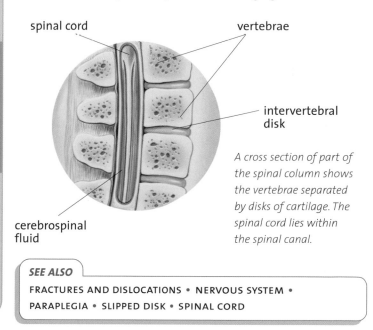

spinal cord

vertebrae

intervertebral disk

cerebrospinal fluid

A cross section of part of the spinal column shows the vertebrae separated by disks of cartilage. The spinal cord lies within the spinal canal.

SEE ALSO

FRACTURES AND DISLOCATIONS • NERVOUS SYSTEM • PARAPLEGIA • SLIPPED DISK • SPINAL CORD

Spinal Cord

The spinal cord, running most of the length of the spinal column, is part of the nervous system. It provides a vital link between the brain and the nerves connected to the rest of the body. There are 31 pairs of spinal nerves, which branch out from the spinal cord to the surface of the body and the muscles.

The spinal cord makes the first analysis of sensations traveling to the brain and acts as a programming station for some basic movements of the limbs. If a person touches something hot, for example, the message is processed before it reaches the brain, producing an instant reflex action so that the hand pulls away. Any further action is dictated by the brain. Some automatic movements, such as those involved in breathing and digestion, are controlled partly by the spinal cord.

Various diseases affect the spinal cord, including poliomyelitis, multiple sclerosis, Lou Gehrig's disease (a type of motor neuron disease), and meningitis.

The spinal cord can also be damaged as a result of injuries to the spinal column.

The spinal nerves control sensations and movement in different areas of the body. If the spinal cord is damaged high in the neck, all of the limbs will be paralyzed and the patient will require help to do many basic tasks, such as eating and dressing.

Q & A

Can ordinary viruses, such as those that cause influenza, cause an infection of the spinal cord?

This can occur, but it is rare.

Are the cells of the spinal cord like brain cells, or are they different?

The nerve cells, or neurons, of the spinal cord are the same as those of the brain. Although some cells are specialized for their particular job (just as some brain cells are), they are essentially the same.

Is the spinal cord always seriously deformed when a baby is born with spina bifida?

No, the spinal cord is not always deformed. There are degrees of severity. It is only in the most severe type of spina bifida that the spinal cord is involved.

brain

spinal cord

31 pairs of spinal nerves branching from spinal cord

Body area controlled by cervical spinal nerves
Body area controlled by thoracic spinal nerves
Body area controlled by lumbar spinal nerves
Body area controlled by sacral spinal nerves

SEE ALSO

MOTOR NEURON DISEASE • NERVOUS SYSTEM • PARAPLEGIA • REFLEXES • SPINAL COLUMN

Sports

Healthy people need exercise, and one of the most enjoyable ways of exercising is to take up some kind of sport. There are so many different sports activities that no matter where people live or what sort of activity they prefer there is certain to be a sport they can take part in and enjoy. Sports do not just keep the body fit and healthy; they are also an enjoyable way of meeting other people and making friends.

Some people take their sports very seriously, spending a great deal of time, effort, and money on them. They may have to travel a long distance to take part or to find the best surroundings and conditions. Others just want some fun and exercise. They will probably look around locally and take up anything that seems enjoyable and convenient.

Joining a team

Many people take part in sports in school or college. The choices may include team games such as baseball, football, and hockey. People who like these games often join clubs where they can continue playing after they finish school. Much of the fun of team games comes from interacting with other people, both

Q & A

Do the warm-up exercises that athletes do really prevent them from getting a stitch in the side when they compete?

The purpose of an athlete's warm-up is to ease muscles into well-oiled working order without overstraining them. Because a stitch originates in the diaphragm, or in the muscles between the ribs, warming up should help prevent it. However, when a stitch occurs because the body is fatigued or suffering from lack of salt, it is not likely that warming up would have made any significant difference.

My brother is a hemophiliac. He wants to play sports, but my mother thinks it would be too dangerous for him. Is she right, or should my brother be allowed to participate in sports?

He can enjoy an active life, but there are certain restrictions. He must avoid contact sports, but he can still swim, run, and play golf, for example.

Running in a relay requires a high level of fitness and skill. The runners need to undergo intensive training so that they can achieve maximum performance.

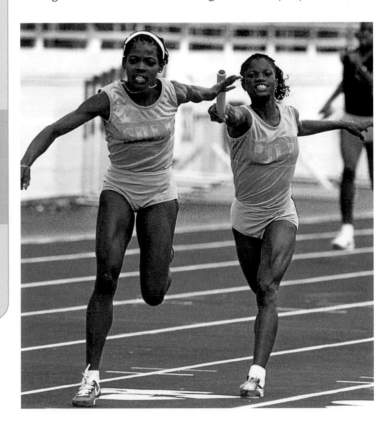

Competitive cycling is an increasingly popular sport in the United States. Whether people are cycling for sport or pleasure, they should always wear a protective helmet.

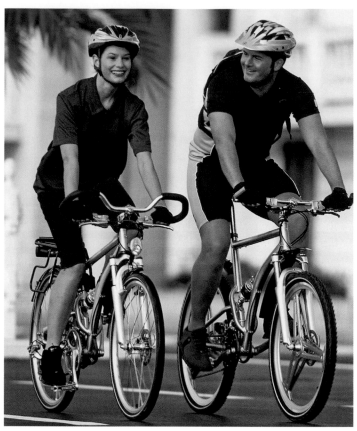

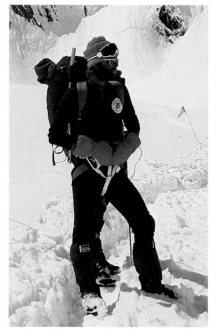

Mountaineering is an exhilarating but potentially dangerous sport that has claimed many lives. It requires fitness and stamina, and only experienced climbers should tackle difficult slopes. Young mountaineers should always be supervised by an expert team leader, even on easy or gentle climbs.

on and off the field. Clubs usually have nonplaying supporters as well, who get a great deal of enjoyment even if they do not get the benefit of exercise.

Many people do not enjoy team sports. They may enjoy games that involve just a few players, such as racquetball or tennis. There are many clubs where these games are played and which cater to all levels, from skilled players to absolute beginners.

Some people prefer track-and-field sports, in which they develop their own abilities as far as possible and then compete against others. Many places have athletic clubs where interested people can get training in such sports. Here, sports are usually taken very seriously, and members spend a great deal of time and effort in improving their fitness and skill.

Types of sports

Not all people are competitive—nor are all sports. Many people meet to walk, run, hike, or bicycle together with no worries about who is fastest or best. These sports have many advantages; they

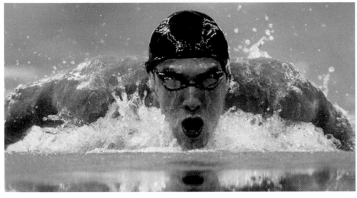

Michael Phelps (b. 1985) set a new record for the most gold medals won at a single Olympics when he won eight gold medals in 2008. Swimming is one of the best forms of exercise for overall fitness. It can be practiced as a competitive sport or simply enjoyed as a group, family, or solitary activity.

require no special training and little equipment, and people can go almost anywhere to carry them out.

Other sports depend on where people live. Those who live near an ocean or lake shore can enjoy water sports, such as swimming, waterskiing, windsurfing, sailing, and sometimes surfing, rowing, or canoeing. Mountain dwellers can take part in climbing and skiing. Some sports such as horseback riding are more common, less expensive, and more enjoyable in the country than in a city. City people have the advantage of skating rinks and sports centers and clubs. Sports are not just for the young. Although serious athletes peak in their twenties, many games allow older people to make up in skill for what they have lost in speed and strength. Sailing and golf are two examples of the sports that can be enjoyed by people who are no longer young in years.

Getting fit

Some sports do people more good than others in terms of fitness. Swimming rates highly; it improves the health of the heart and lungs and the suppleness of the joints, and it builds muscle power. All strenuous activities that make people puff and pant are good exercise for the heart and lungs, including ice skating, skiing, hockey, football, tennis, racquetball, rowing, brisk jogging, and cycling. Gymnastics and horseback riding are among the sports that make the joints supple. However, no sport will do much good unless people take part regularly and sensibly.

Warming up

Before starting any sports, people should do warm-up exercises to prepare the muscles and avoid strains. It is best to wear the right clothes, including special shoes and protective headgear where necessary, and make sure that any equipment is safe and in good working order. Many sports, particularly the most exciting ones, can be dangerous even for experts, and the best way to avoid accidents is to learn from a professional teacher.

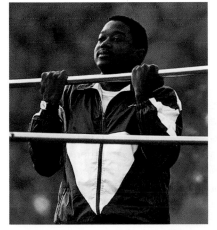

This man is lifting his body using a metal bar. Whatever sports people take part in, they need to enjoy training to keep at peak fitness levels.

SEE ALSO

EXERCISE • HEART • JOGGING • MUSCLE • PHYSICAL FITNESS • SPORTS INJURIES • SPRAINS AND STRAINS

Sports Injuries

Almost every sport involves some risk of injury, from trivial cuts and bruises to more serious damage. Perhaps the most hazardous sports are those involving high speed (such as automobile racing, motorcycle racing, and skiing) and those carried out in dangerous places (such as mountaineering). Body contact sports (such as football and boxing) can also pose dangers. Some people are hurt accidentally by equipment; for example, being spiked by a fellow athlete's track shoes is a common injury.

Head injuries

Head injuries are a risk in contact sports such as boxing, where repeated blows to the head can cause long-lasting damage as the brain is knocked around inside the skull. Other sports are potentially dangerous. They include football and wrestling, as well as automobile, motorcycle, and bike racing. Horseback riding is another sport in which serious head injuries, fractures, and dislocations can occur.

Potential brain damage

All head injuries are potentially serious, because they can cause skull fractures, concussion, contusion, or internal bleeding. If a head injury is not correctly diagnosed and treated, headaches, loss of memory, and even permanent brain damage can result. However slight an injury seems, it is always best to get a doctor's opinion. A preventive measure, such as wearing a protective helmet, provides the best safeguard.

Muscle damage and tendon injuries

Most often, a sports injury follows the overuse of some part of the body. Muscle injuries are very

This rock climber is using the proper safety equipment and wearing a protective hard hat. Young climbers should always be supervised, and only experienced climbers should tackle difficult slopes.

Soccer players often receive ankle injuries as a result of careless tackling.

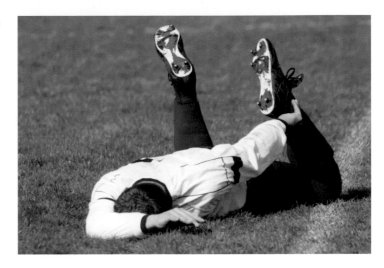

common and usually involve a rupture of some of the muscle fibers. These injuries are described in various ways: as a pull, a tear, or a strain. Soccer players frequently suffer injuries to the thigh muscles, calf muscles, and ankles; sprinters may damage the hamstrings at the back of the thigh.

The Achilles tendon above the heel is commonly injured by runners, hurdlers, and long jumpers; tendons (the fibrous cords that join muscle and bone) can also become inflamed through overuse. Rowers and racket players, for example, are at risk of inflammation of the wrist and elbow tendons. Such injuries should never be taken lightly.

Torn ligaments and tendons require just as long to heal as fractures of the bones, and inflamed tendons may need several weeks of rest from sports until the pain subsides. Even then, the return to sporting activity should be taken gradually to avoid further damage.

Knee and ankle injuries

Knee joints and ankle joints are particularly easy to injure, and once they are damaged, they are prone to weakness later on. Apart from dislocation, one of the most frequent injuries to the knee is a torn cartilage, which is very painful and makes movement of the knee difficult. Hairline fractures (shin splints) often occur in the shins of runners who overtrain on hard, jarring surfaces, such as pavements.

Avoiding injury

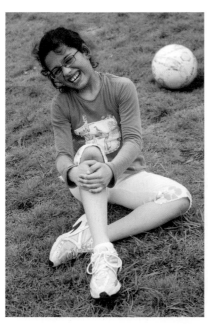

This girl fell down and hurt her knee while chasing after a ball.

Most sports injuries can be avoided through a mixture of fitness training, adequate preparation for the particular sport, and

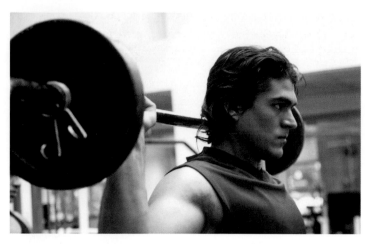

Weight lifting is an excellent activity for keeping the muscles in shape. However, it is important to receive instruction first to avoid causing unnecessary injuries.

common sense. Conditioning exercises are very important, particularly at the beginning of the sports season, when fitness levels may not be up to standard.

If people are taking part in serious or competitive sports, they should be guided by their coach, who will make sure that they have the appropriate training exercises before being allowed to play. He or she will also insist on proper stretching and warm-up routines before people undertake any strenuous sports activity. If a suitable warm-up is omitted or not properly carried out, many injuries can occur, such as strained elbows, damaged knee joints, pulled muscles, and stress fractures.

Treating sports injuries

With most sports injuries, the first thing to do is to reduce the pain and swelling in the affected areas. A coach or a doctor can advise on further treatment, which usually involves resting the injured part for a few weeks or even longer. Sometimes physical therapy may be necessary.

Apart from minor injuries, all other sports injuries should be examined by an expert. If there is any doubt, and particularly if pain is experienced, people with sports injuries should visit the emergency room.

Proceeding with caution

If people have been out of action because of illness or injury, they must regain their fitness levels before they resume play. Too many people are tempted to make up for lost time by playing too vigorously and too soon after an injury has occurred. This action can lead to permanent damage or chronic weakness in the injured part.

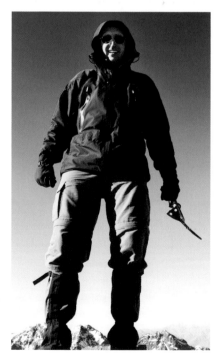

Mountaineering is an exhilarating but potentially dangerous sport that has claimed many lives.

SEE ALSO

BLACK EYE • BRUISES • FRACTURES AND DISLOCATIONS • HAMSTRING INJURIES • ICE THERAPY • JOINTS • KNEE • MUSCLE • MUSCLE DISEASES AND DISORDERS • PHYSICAL FITNESS • PHYSICAL THERAPY • SPORTS • SPRAINS AND STRAINS • TENDON • TENNIS ELBOW

Sprains and Strains

Q & A

What is the best type of bandage to use for treating a sprain?

The aim is to give the joint firm support while it heals, but it should not be completely immobilized. Some form of elasticized bandage is therefore required. An ordinary cotton bandage gives too little support, but crepe, webbing, and elastic bandages are all suitable. The bandage must be tight enough to be effective but not so tight that it interferes with the circulation; impairing the circulation could cause gangrene.

My friend recommended a massage to treat my sprain. Is that a good idea?

Perhaps. Gentle massage can be started when the immediate effects of the injury have worn off, usually on the second or third day. The area will be very tender, so only light pressure should be applied.

Sprains are common injuries that happen to almost everyone at some time. They are the result of twisting or wrenching a joint farther than it can normally move. As a result, the ligaments that hold the joint in position are stretched and some of the fibers are torn. The blood vessels in the area are usually torn, too. Strains are less serious; fibers in the muscles are stretched or torn.

People often sprain an ankle if they trip or sprain a wrist as the result of a fall. Larger joints, such as the knee or hip, may be sprained during sports. A sprained neck can occur as a result of whiplash injury in an automobile accident, although such injuries have become less common since safety belts and head restrainers were introduced.

The obvious signs of a sprain are sudden, severe pain from the stretched or torn ligaments around the joint and swelling and bruising caused by bleeding in the area around it. This pain becomes much worse if the injured person tries to move or use the joint or put weight on it.

Strained shoulder, leg, and wrist muscles and turned ankles are common sports injuries. The most frequent strains affect less active people and occur in the lower back as a result of picking up a heavy or awkward object. Learning how to lift and carry things properly can prevent back injury and pain. When lifting something heavy, it is best to keep the back straight and bend the knees, letting them take the weight.

Rest, painkillers, and heat treatment will help most strains. Any injury more serious than a minor sprain should be examined by a doctor, just in case a joint has been fractured.

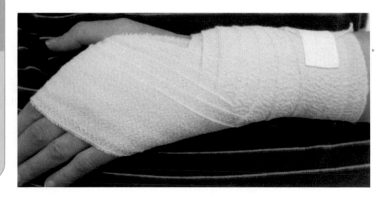

After first aid to help reduce the pain and swelling of a sprained wrist, a doctor will usually wrap the hand and wrist in an elasticized bandage to support the wrist and prevent further injury.

SEE ALSO

BACKACHE • EXERCISE • FRACTURES AND DISLOCATIONS • HIP • ICE THERAPY • JOGGING • KNEE • LEG • LIGAMENTS • MUSCLE • PAIN • SHOULDER • SPORTS INJURIES

Stroke

When a person has a stroke, the normal blood supply to part of the brain is interrupted. A clot may form in one of the brain's arteries and block it (cerebral thrombosis). A clot or piece of artery wall from somewhere else in the body may be carried in the bloodstream to the brain and cause a blockage there (cerebral embolism). The most serious types of strokes are caused by an artery that bleeds into the brain (cerebral hemorrhage).

When the blood supply to part of the brain is cut off, that area of the brain suddenly stops working. The patient's symptoms will depend on what functions this area controlled. A stroke may cause weakness or paralysis down one side of the body, loss of sight on one side, or loss of speech or understanding. If a very large area of the brain is affected, the patient may die.

However, there are many cross-connections between neighboring areas of the brain, so the area of damage is not usually very great. The brain has spare areas that, in time, may be able to take over some of the work done by the damaged area. Thus, stroke patients may recover almost completely after a while, with physical therapy and speech therapy when necessary.

Strokes are caused by disease of the arteries and high blood pressure (which can weaken the artery walls). Smokers and people with diabetes or a high level of cholesterol in the blood are at greater risk.

Q & A

My grandfather has just had a stroke and can't speak. Will his speech return?

Yes, it is very likely that his ability to speak will come back, at least to some extent. Sometimes, people are unable to speak at all in the first few days after a stroke, but they later recover almost completely.

My uncle had a bad heart attack and then a few weeks later had a stroke that paralyzed his left side. Was this connected with his heart attack?

After a heart attack, blood clots may form on the inside wall of the chamber of the heart. Occasionally, part of a clot can dislodge and block off one of the brain's blood vessels, thus producing a stroke. Patients who have had very serious heart attacks can be given anticoagulant drugs to help prevent this.

This stroke patient has aphasia. She has difficulty in understanding words as well as speaking them. Here she attempts to name familiar objects. In time, and with good therapy, she should recover her use of language skills.

SEE ALSO

BLOOD PRESSURE • CHOLESTEROL • CIRCULATORY SYSTEM • DIABETES • DIET • DIETING • EXERCISE • HEART ATTACK • PHYSICAL THERAPY

Sugars

Sugar is an important carbohydrate food. It suppli[...] with energy, and its sweetness is used to enhanc[...] of many foods and candies. All green plants mak[...] chemical name of sugar is sucrose. White sugar is the same as brown sugar except that it is simply more refined.

During digestion, sugars and starch are broken down into simpler sugars called fructose and glucose. Other kinds of sugars are lactose (present in milk) and maltose (present in corn). These simple sugars are absorbed into the body and used as fuel to provide energy for all metabolic processes. Some glucose is diverted to the liver, converted to glycogen, and stored. When instant energy is required, the liver converts some of the stored glycogen into glucose and releases it into the bloodstream. If there is a temporary lack of carbohydrates, the liver is able to synthesize glucose from fats and proteins.

All the cells in the body use sugar as a source of energy. The blood contains about 0.1 percent glucose, which supplies energy to the various body tissues, especially to the brain.

Blood sugar, insulin, and diabetes

Hormones control the amount of sugar in the blood. The most important of these hormones is insulin. Too little insulin, or a total lack of it, leads to high concentrations of blood sugar. This

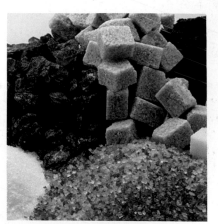

condition is called diabetes. Overproduction of insulin leads to too little sugar in the blood, producing a condition called hypoglycemia, which quickly impairs the function of the brain. People suffering from hypoglycemia learn to recognize the onset of symptoms and eat a sugar-rich food to avert an attack.

Q & A

Do glucose tablets and drinks provide instant energy?

No. Glucose is the fuel that gives the body energy, but it does not instantly provide energy. Glucose is stored in the liver and muscles as glycogen until it is required. The amount of glucose present in the blood is tiny, and more is added from the glycogen store when blood sugar levels drop. All carbohydrates convert to glucose, so there is no need to take glucose tablets and drinks.

Why do diabetics have to restrict their sugar intake?

A diabetic diet consists of a controlled amount of all carbohydrates. Diabetes is caused by the inability of the body to control the amount of sugar in the blood, so the diet aims to provide the patient with the exact amount of required carbohydrates.

Most sugar is produced using the juice extracted from sugarcane. Brown sugar is generally less refined than white sugar and contains trace minerals and organic substances. Some brown sugars, however, are just white sugars that have been artificially colored.

SEE ALSO

APPETITE · BASAL METABOLISM · BODY SYSTEMS · CALORIES · CARBOHYDRATES · DIABETES · DIET · DIETING · DIGESTIVE SYSTEM · FATS · FOOD ADDITIVES · FOOD AND NUTRITION · JUNK FOOD · OBESITY · PROTEIN · WEIGHT CONTROL

Sunburn

Sunburn is now less common than it used to be. People are gradually taking notice of doctors' warnings that too much sun is a health risk. Sunburn is very uncomfortable, painful, and dangerous. Repeated sunburn can damage the skin permanently, and skin cancer is most likely to occur in fair-skinned people who have spent a long time in strong sunlight.

Sunburn is caused by ultraviolet rays from the sun, which damage the outer layer of the skin. These rays stimulate the skin to produce a pigment called melanin, which darkens the skin to provide protection and acts as a filter for the ultraviolet rays. Sunburn occurs when there is not enough pigment produced by the cells to filter the sun's rays.

Dangers of sunburn

Sunburn is not felt until a little while after it happens. The first signs are redness and a feeling of burning caused by an increase of the blood supply to the skin. Sunburned legs and arms may swell painfully, and the victim may develop a headache and fever and may vomit. Heat exhaustion may also occur. Blisters may develop, and the surface layer of skin may peel off.

Many people think that a suntan is attractive, but repeated sun exposure over time makes the skin heavily wrinkled and

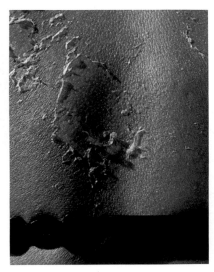

leathery. Patchy areas of skin pigmentation and wartlike lumps (solar keratoses) may develop.

Sunburn can be treated with soothing lotions and ointments, but it is much more sensible not to get it in the first place. When out in the sun, people should use sunscreen with a high sun protection factor (SPF) to cover exposed areas of the body. Otherwise, it is best to keep out of the sun or keep the skin covered.

Q & A

I am fair-skinned and my friend is dark. Why can she spend a long time in the sun without burning while I cannot?

Being fair-skinned means that you have little pigment in your skin. Your friend has more pigment and can also make more than you when exposed to sunlight. You will burn easily, because your skin cannot produce enough protective pigment, but it is dangerous for *anyone* to spend a long time in the sun.

My family is planning a vacation to the Caribbean. What can I do to reduce the risk of sunburn?

You could have a course of ultraviolet ray therapy beforehand, to increase your pigmentation. You could also use a sunscreen preparation that filters out the sun's stronger rays, allowing a slow tan to develop. The best way to protect yourself is to stay out of the sun altogether.

A suntan does not prevent sunburn. Once the pigment-producing cells have been saturated with ultraviolet light, further exposure causes burning, unattractive peeling skin, and long-term skin damage.

SEE ALSO

AGING • BLISTERS • CIRCULATORY SYSTEM • HEAT SICKNESS • PAIN • SKIN • SWEAT

Sweat

Perspiration, or sweat, plays a vitally important part in keeping the body at the right temperature. A small amount of sweat is constantly released onto the skin. As it evaporates, it cools down the body. If people get hot, they perspire more heavily, and this process cools them more quickly. If the body did not lose heat like this, people would suffer from heat stroke and die.

Sweat consists of water, salt, and, in some cases, organic matter. There are two kinds of sweat glands, apocrine and eccrine. Apocrine glands are present only on the hairy areas of the body, such as the armpits and groin. Sweat from apocrine glands contains some of the cells from the gland linings, whereas eccrine gland sweat contains only water and salt. At puberty, the apocrine sweat glands develop. They produce increased underarm sweating and the odor that comes from sweat. A woman's milk-producing mammary glands are a type of apocrine gland.

Most people produce about 1 pint (0.5 l) of sweat every day. In very hot conditions, people may produce a lot more, and they need to drink a lot of water and take salt tablets to replace what has been lost. When people have a fever, the body temperature rises, and they perspire noticeably. Episodes of perspiring, particularly at night, can be a symptom of some types of illnesses. Anyone with a fever should drink plenty of fluids.

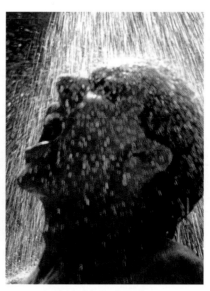

The organic matter in sweat is broken down by bacteria on the skin surface to produce an unpleasant smell, particularly under the armpits. This body odor can be controlled by showering daily and by wearing clean clothes every day. Deodorants just mask the odor; antiperspirants reduce pore size or clog the pores to retard perspiration.

Q & A

Is perspiration just another word for sweat?

Yes, but perspiration generally describes moderate sweating—a steady production of sweat that does not form into heavy droplets.

Why do some people seem to sweat more than others?

The mechanism of sweating is controlled by the nerves and is affected by both a person's excitability and the state of the skin's blood vessels. Heavier people have to sweat more to cool themselves off, and anxious people sweat more because their nerves are more active.

Is there anything I can do to stop my feet from sweating?

The short answer is no. The soles of your feet, like the palms of your hands, have many hundreds of sweat glands that are important for controlling your body temperature.

Frequent showering or bathing helps prevent perspiration from causing body odor. In hot weather, a lukewarm shower helps to keep the body cool and is extremely refreshing.

SEE ALSO

DRINKING WATER • GLANDS • HEAT SICKNESS • NERVOUS SYSTEM • SALT • SKIN

Tendon

A tendon, also called a sinew, is a very tough band of fibrous tissue that connects a muscle to a part of the body, usually a bone, so that it can carry out movements. Tendons are extensions of muscles; their fibers fuse with the connective tissue that covers the bone.

Several tendons are located close to the surface of the body and can be easily felt. An example is the hamstring tendon at the back of the knee. Others can be seen in the backs of the hands and the soles of the feet. Tendons run inside sheaths at the points where they cross or are in contact with other structures. Each sheath is a double-walled sleeve, with the space between the walls filled with lubricating fluid. Repeated movements may cause the fluid to run dry. Rest is essential until this fluid builds up again; otherwise inflammation, called tendonitis, may result.

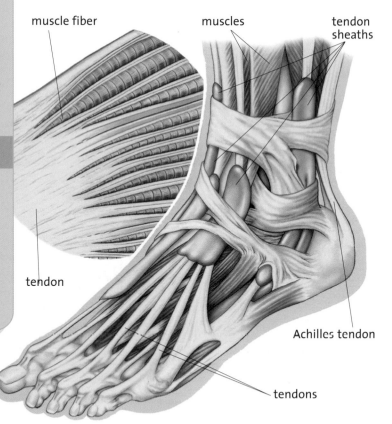

muscle fiber

muscles

tendon sheaths

tendon

Achilles tendon

tendons

The muscle fibers merge to form tendons that are attached to bones. Where the tendons cross each other or other structures, they are protected by a fluid-filled sheath.

SEE ALSO

MUSCLE • MUSCLE DISEASES AND DISORDERS • SPORTS INJURIES

Tennis Elbow

Tennis elbow is inflammation of the tendon where it attaches to the bone at the outer side of the elbow. The tendon links the muscle in the upper arm to the bone in the forearm and can become damaged owing to repeated use of the forearm, such as playing backhand shots in tennis. Other types of activities, such as excessive use of a screwdriver (where the wrist and forearm are vigorously worked), can also cause tennis elbow. The tendon becomes pulled, and small tears may occur, leading to pain and tenderness in the area.

Symptoms and treatments

When someone suffers from tennis elbow, the elbow looks normal, and bending and straightening the arm are painless and unrestricted. However, there is fairly constant pain and tenderness experienced in the elbow region. In severe cases, the pain may be felt over a much wider area, often extending well over the back of the forearm. The pain is made worse by actions such as turning a stiff doorknob or unscrewing a jar top.

Most cases of tennis elbow settle with physical therapy, ice packs, exercises to stretch and strengthen the affected muscles, ultrasound treatment, and the avoidance of any activity that causes pain. Some people have found acupuncture and heat treatment helpful.

If these actions fail, a doctor may inject a corticosteroid with a local anesthetic into the affected area. In rare cases, surgery may be needed. If the condition is caused by playing sports, expert coaching on technique may be necessary.

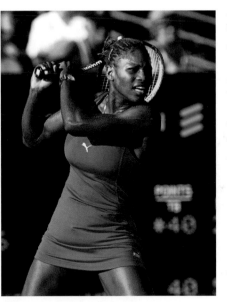

Q & A

If I had tennis elbow, how would I be able to recognize it?

You would have a dull ache around the elbow area and upper side of the forearm, with a particularly tender spot on the bump that can be felt on the upper side of the elbow when the forearm is placed across the chest. Typing, using a squash or tennis racket, or even picking up heavy objects may be painful.

How soon can one resume playing tennis after tennis elbow?

That depends on how serious the injury was; you should seek your doctor's advice. The symptoms vary from person to person. In mild cases, it may take only a few days until the pain and stiffness subside, and then you can resume the sport gradually. More serious cases may take longer. If the tenderness returns whenever you play, consult your doctor as soon as possible.

Serena Williams follows through after a backhand shot. Tennis players can suffer from tennis elbow, usually as a result of overuse of the muscles and tendons used to hit a backhand shot.

SEE ALSO

ACUPUNCTURE • ELBOW • ICE THERAPY • MUSCLE • PAIN • PHYSICAL THERAPY • SPORTS INJURIES • TENDON

Tiredness

Q & A

How can you tell the difference between a person who is lazy and a person who is tired because of an illness?

In general, the lazy person is able to find a huge amount of energy to do what he or she enjoys doing, whereas a truly exhausted person cannot summon up enthusiasm for anything.

My grandmother, who is 81, seems very feeble and tired lately. She thinks this condition is due to her age and won't consult her doctor. Is she right?

Although there is some loss of energy in old age, it should be slight and gradual. Anything more should not be accepted as normal or inevitable and should be investigated, because it can often be helped. Anemia and inadequate nutrition may be due to a reluctance to buy and cook nutritious food; this problem is common in older people. Your family should continue trying to persuade your grandmother to see a doctor about her tiredness.

Babies cry when they are tired. They may also become so overtired that they are unable to sleep and need to be calmed.

Most people feel tired after a day's hard work or exercise. They may also feel tired during the day if they have slept badly the previous night. Usually, a good night's sleep is all that is needed to make the tiredness disappear. However, tiredness can also be a sign of illness. A person with persistent tiredness may have daytime sleepiness and a lack of energy, loss of motivation, poor concentration, difficulty in making decisions, and depression.

Often, tiredness is due to a combination of causes. Nine in 100 people with tiredness have a physical disease; about 75 in 100 people have an emotional condition. The most common cause of abnormal tiredness is an infection.

Sometimes, tiredness is an early warning of an illness; people often feel tired for a day or two before developing influenza or the common cold. Tiredness is also the main symptom of some mild infectious diseases, such as rubella (German measles) and infectious mononucleosis. Diseases such as measles, chicken pox, and influenza often leave people feeling tired and run down.

Two other common causes of tiredness are anemia and hormone diseases (including lack of thyroid hormone and diabetes). However, tiredness can also have mental or emotional causes, including boredom, anxiety, and depression. Severe, long-term, debilitating tiredness may be a symptom of chronic fatigue syndrome. This condition does not readily respond to treatment, but many sufferers find they improve over time.

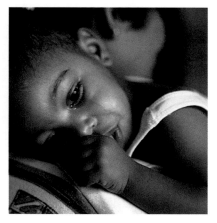

Tiredness, fatigue, and lethargy
Tiredness is also sometimes known as fatigue (weariness or exhaustion caused by exertion). Lethargy, however, usually means an indifference to events, a general lack of inclination to take part in any activity, or an abnormal lack of energy.

SEE ALSO

ANEMIA • CHRONIC FATIGUE SYNDROME • DIABETES • EXERCISE • LETHARGY • REST AND RELAXATION

Vegetarianism

Vegetarians are people who do not eat meat. They may dislike the idea of animals being killed to provide meat, find the taste of meat unpleasant, or feel healthier on a vegetarian diet. Doctors may suggest a vegetarian diet for certain medical conditions. Some religions and spiritual sects forbid eating meat, and certain Indian and African communities eat no meat.

Many vegetarians do eat dairy products, such as milk and eggs. People following a macrobiotic diet eat foods based on whole grains, cereals, some vegetables, and occasionally fish. Vegans eat no animal products of any kind. People considering a vegetarian diet should take a responsible approach to ensure that they have a regular intake of essential vitamins and minerals, because strict vegetarians can lack some of these essential substances in their diet.

A properly balanced vegetarian diet can contain all the nutrition people need to keep healthy. It also has the advantage of being low in saturated fats (which can cause heart disease) and high in fiber. Eggs and cheese provide protein, but vegans can also get enough protein by combining cereals, nuts, legumes, potatoes, and oil seeds. Some vitamins (including vitamin B and vitamin D) are not present in plants, so vegans should take vitamin supplements to provide them.

In terms of land use, it is more economical to grow crops than to graze animals for slaughter. If less grain were used to raise animals, more would be available for humans to eat. About 50 percent of the world cereal crop is fed to animals, and it takes 10 tons of vegetable protein to yield just one ton of animal protein.

10 acres (4 hectares) of land feed the following number of people:

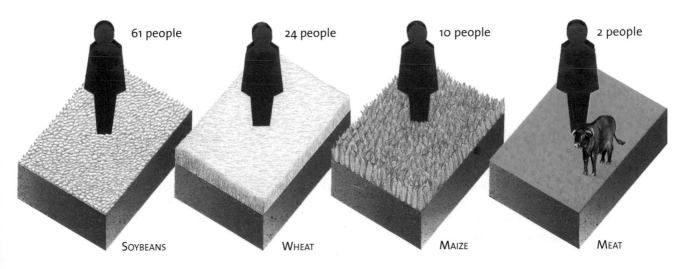

61 people — SOYBEANS
24 people — WHEAT
10 people — MAIZE
2 people — MEAT

SEE ALSO

DIET • DIGESTIVE SYSTEM • FOOD AND NUTRITION • MINERALS • NUTRITIONAL DISEASES • PROTEIN • VITAMINS

Vitamins

To function efficiently, the body needs vitamins. These chemical substances are involved in the processes of repair and maintenance of the body's tissues. Some vitamins are made by the body—for example, the skin can make vitamin D from sunlight—but people get most of the vitamins they require from food. A balanced diet should provide all the essential vitamins.

Many nutritional diseases are caused by lack of vitamins in the diet. All the B vitamins are necessary for the proper operation of various enzymes. Vitamin C is required for the production of healthy collagen (the structural protein present in bones, ligaments, and tendons). Vitamin C is also a powerful antioxidant that mops up damaging chemical groups called free radicals.

Naming vitamins

Vitamins are generally known by letters of the alphabet, and sometimes by other names. The main vitamins are A, B, C, D, E, and K. Of these, A, D, E, and K are fat-soluble and can be stored in the body, but vitamins B and C are water-soluble and cannot.

Deficiency diseases

Most people in developed countries get all the vitamins they need in their everyday food. The exceptions are elderly people, alcoholics, and those who cannot afford appropriate food. Some people have deficiency diseases because their bodies cannot absorb the vitamins they eat. Deficiency diseases still occur in poor parts of the world where the diet is inadequate or where food is scarce. Perhaps the most common vitamin deficiency is vitamin A (which causes eye problems). The body can make vitamin A from fresh vegetables but they are in short supply in developing countries. Hundreds of thousands of children go blind every year from vitamin A deficiency. Their corneas soften, melt, and split, and infection destroys their eyes.

Many people throughout the developed world take vitamin supplements in the belief that vitamins will keep them healthy, although everyone who eats a properly balanced diet should have sufficient vitamins from the food that is eaten. Indeed, extra intake of certain vitamins can be harmful. However, vitamins C and E are known to protect the body against free radicals, which are thought to be implicated in many diseases and are involved in the deposition of harmful cholesterol in the artery walls. Numerous clinical trials have shown that people who have an above-average intake of the antioxidant vitamins C and E also have a lower-than-average incidence of these diseases. For these reasons, millions of people now take daily vitamin supplements.

Q & A

What are vitamins and how important are they?

Vitamins are organic substances present in minute amounts in food. They help make the body work. Because they cannot be made in the body, vitamins must be obtained from the diet or from sunshine. A person requires only small amounts, but vitamins are nevertheless essential to normal metabolism.

I have very low energy levels. Have I got a vitamin deficiency?

It is most unlikely that a person on a normal diet would suffer a vitamin deficiency. The only time extra vitamins should be taken is when you are on an abnormal or restricted diet.

Can taking too many vitamins be harmful?

Taking too much vitamin A and D can be harmful. Too much vitamin A can result in fragile bones, enlargement of the liver and spleen, and loss of appetite. Vitamin D overdose can cause vomiting, headache, weight loss, and calcium deposits in the kidneys and arteries.

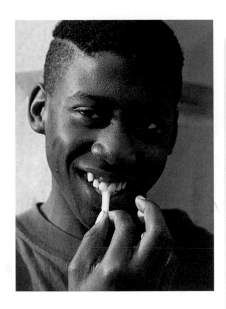

Junk food may be very tasty, but it is deficient in essential nutrients, especially vitamins. For this reason, it should not form a major part of the daily diet.

LIMEYS

Vitamins were discovered in the early twentieth century, but hundreds of years ago people realized that eating certain foods helped keep them healthy, even if they did not know why. In 1753, a British naval surgeon described how lemons, limes, and other citrus fruits could prevent sailors at sea from getting a disease called scurvy, which caused spongy gums, loose teeth, and bleeding into the skin. This is why British sailors came to be nicknamed "limeys." Now people know that scurvy is caused by a lack of vitamin C, which is present in fresh vegetables and especially in citrus fruits.

VITAMINS AND VITAMIN DEFICIENCY

Vitamin	Deficiency symptoms	Good sources
A (retinol)	Night blindness, growth retardation, aggravation of lung diseases, rough dry skin, and blindness	Liver, fish, dairy products, eggs, carrots, green vegetables (particularly spinach), and margarine
B_1 (thiamine)	Memory loss, appetite loss, digestive disturbances, fatigue, nervousness, and beriberi	Whole-grain cereals, fortified breakfast cereals, meat, milk, green vegetables, brewer's yeast, wheat germ, and yeast extract
B_2 (riboflavin)	Corner-of-mouth cracks and sores, dizziness, light sensitivity, and eye lesions	Milk, organ meats (particularly liver), eggs, and green vegetables
B_3 (niacin; also known as PP, which stands for pellagra-preventing)	Appetite loss, headaches, depression, memory impairment, nervous disorders, and pellagra with symptoms of dark, scaly skin	Lean meat, liver, legumes, fortified breakfast cereals, bread, eggs, and milk products
B_5 (pantothenic acid)	Very rare	Most foods
B_6 (pyridoxine)	Low levels sometimes found in women who are pregnant or on the Pill; associated with fatigue and depression, irritation of the lips, and dry skin	Most foods (particularly meat, vegetables, yeast, cereals, bread, milk products, and eggs)
B_9 (folic acid)	Digestive disturbance, growth problems, anemia, and possibly spina bifida	Most green leafy vegetables, organ meats, legumes, and bread
B_{12} (cyanocobalamin)	Fatigue, memory impairment, pernicious anemia, and degeneration of nerve cells	Dairy and animal products (particularly liver)
C (ascorbic acid)	Anemia, bleeding gums, and scurvy	Fresh fruits (particularly citrus and black currants), vegetables, and potatoes
D (calciferol)	Bone deformity (rickets and osteomalacia) and poor teeth	Cod liver oil, egg yolk, fatty fish, butter and fortified margarine; also made by the body in sunlight
E (tocopherol)	Hemolytic anemia in premature infants	Most foods, especially cereals, eggs, nuts, wheat germ, and vegetable oils
K (phylloquinone)	Impairment of blood-clotting process	Dark green vegetables and liver; also made by bacteria in the intestine

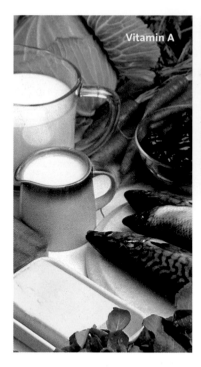

Vitamin A

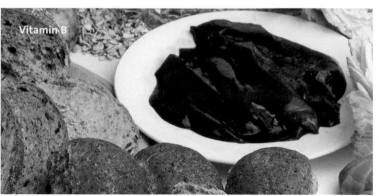

Vitamin B

Vitamin A

Vitamin A is present in liver, fish oils, dairy products, and egg yolks. The body can also make vitamin A from the substance carotene, which is present in carrots and green vegetables. Vitamin A plays a part in bone and tooth formation, in maintaining the membranes that line the body tubes, in general growth, and in keeping the tissues of the eyes healthy. Vitamin A can be stored in the liver. A deficiency of Vitamin A may cause night blindness, poor skin, and poor bone growth.

A balanced diet, rich in fresh fruits and vegetables, provides all the vitamins the body needs to stay healthy.

Vitamin B complex

The vitamin B complex is a group of vitamins. Vitamin B_1 is also called thiamine. It is needed to keep the brain, nerves, and muscles working. Vitamin B_2, (riboflavin), vitamin B_3 (niacin), and vitamin B_6 help the body break down food for energy, and vitamins B_9 (folic acid) and B_{12} (cyanocobalamin) are essential for making red blood cells. The B vitamins are present in liver and meat, and some are present in nuts and vegetables. The body cannot store B vitamins, so people need to eat them regularly. Lack of B vitamins causes disorders of the heart and nervous system and diseases such as pellagra, anemia, and beriberi.

Vitamin C

Vitamin C is an antioxidant with many valuable properties. It plays an important part in growth and healing and strengthens the immune system. It is present in fruits (especially citrus fruits) and vegetables. Vitamin C cannot be stored in the body, so if people eat more than they need, the excess is excreted in the urine. For this reason, it is important to eat vitamin C–rich foods daily to restore the body's supplies.

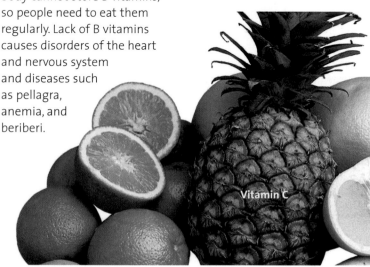

Vitamin C

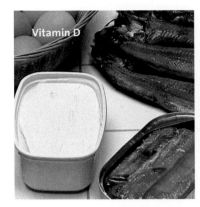

Vitamin D

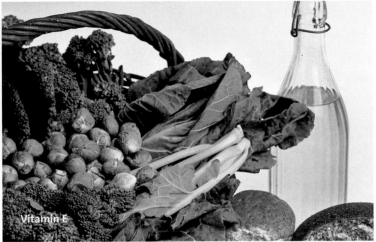

Vitamin E

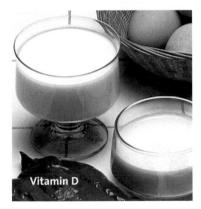

Vitamin D

Vitamin D

Vitamin D helps people absorb calcium and phosphorus and build up a healthy bone structure. It is especially important for babies and young children, because their bodies are growing very fast. The body can make vitamin D from sunlight, but it is also present in oily fish, eggs, and dairy products. People with fair skin make more vitamin D than those with dark skin. Without vitamin D, children suffer from rickets (bone deformities as a result of inadequate supplies of calcium and phosphorus) and poor teeth.

Vitamin E

Like vitamin C, vitamin E is a powerful antioxidant. It is fat-soluble and functions in the fatty cell membranes to help protect them against free radicals. It is present in most foods, particularly vegetable oils, whole-grain cereals, dark green vegetables, and wheat germ. Deficiency can cause muscular problems and may also lead to fertility problems.

Vitamin K

Vitamin K plays an important part in the clotting of blood. Dark green vegetables, potatoes, wheat germ, cheese, liver, and eggs are good sources. Vitamin K can be made by the action of bacteria in the intestines. Although most people get enough vitamin K, deficiency may occur in those people with liver disorders, malabsorption, and chronic diarrhea.

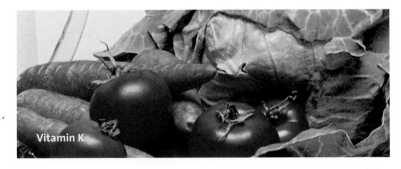

Vitamin K

SEE ALSO

ANEMIA • DIET • DIETING • FOOD AND NUTRITION • HEALTH FOODS • MALNUTRITION • MINERALS • NUTRITIONAL DISEASES • SCURVY

Weight Control

Q & A

I want to lose weight, and several of my friends have suggested that I should join their yoga class. Can I really lose weight by taking up yoga exercise?

Yoga alone may not cause you to shed many pounds, but you should look and feel more trim, because yoga exercises firm and tone the muscles. Yoga postures firm up the abdomen, upper arms, and thighs, which are prone to flabbiness if you are dieting.

Should I use diet pills to try to lose weight?

Doctors agree that the best way to lose weight is to eat less and exercise regularly.

I am overweight, and nothing I've tried in order to lose the weight has worked. Could I have a problem with my adrenal glands?

If your excess weight is distributed evenly, the answer is no. There is only one disease of the adrenals (Cushing's syndrome) that gives rise to obesity and it is extremely rare.

Measuring a patient's weight is a standard part of any medical examination, because weight is often a clue to someone's general state of health. People who are overweight put an extra strain on their body, in particular on their heart. They need to lose weight to maintain their health.

Weight can be lost by dieting sensibly—eating no more than the body needs, while ensuring that it gets essential nourishment—and increasing exercise levels.

Compulsive overeating

Now recognized as an illness, compulsive overeating is a major cause of obesity, together with emotional unhappiness. Many people are secret food addicts who overeat to cover up their anxieties. For them, food offers comfort and security. It is mostly women who are driven to compulsive overeating, often in binges that are followed by drastic purges. Although the risks to mental and physical health are considerable, such people are often unable to help themselves. Psychotherapy or organizations such as Overeaters Anonymous can help find the underlying causes of the compulsion and help people to control their weight sensibly.

Dangers of being underweight

Being underweight can also be unhealthy. It makes people easily tired and less resistant to infection, and it is often a sign that

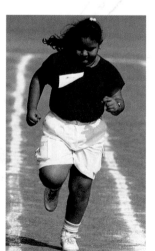

something is wrong. Some people lose weight when they are worried or upset, but loss of weight can also be one of the first signs of illness. People who find that they are more than a few pounds underweight or who are losing weight for no obvious reason should see a doctor. Tests can show if there is an underlying problem, and treatment can be started immediately.

Many obese children find reducing weight enjoying and rewarding. Taking part in sports makes them fitter and increases their self-esteem.

SEE ALSO

ANOREXIA AND BULIMIA • **DIET** • **DIETING** • **EXERCISE** • **FOOD AND NUTRITION** • **OBESITY** • **PHYSICAL FITNESS** • **YOGA**

Yoga

Yoga is a series of exercises or postures that relax the mind and the body and emphasize harmonious coordination of movement, stretching, and breathing. Yoga also helps tone muscles and stimulate blood circulation.

The exercises are intended to work on the whole body. They are performed slowly, gracefully, and thoughtfully. Each posture is held for a period of time to give the muscles a chance to derive the maximum benefit from the position.

Special breathing techniques are used in conjunction with yoga exercises. The basis of yoga breathing is a deeply indrawn breath through the nose, which first expands the abdomen, then the rib cage, and then the chest.

Yoga is an ideal exercise for people of all ages. Because there are no quick or jerky movements, it is suitable for young children and elderly men and women. Yoga is also good for teenagers and younger people, because it helps develop grace, poise, and concentration. Mental tranquillity is another benefit of yoga. Most people say that they feel both refreshed and relaxed after a session of yoga. Although it requires practice to master the exercises, even beginners soon experience feelings of well-being after a couple of yoga sessions.

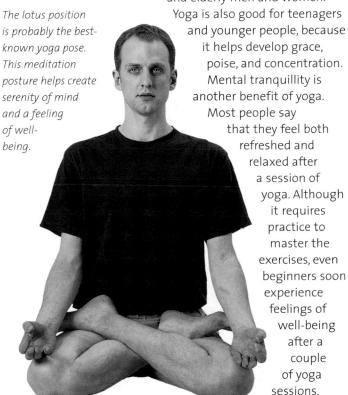

The lotus position is probably the best-known yoga pose. This meditation posture helps create serenity of mind and a feeling of well-being.

SEE ALSO

AEROBICS • ALEXANDER TECHNIQUE • CIRCULATORY SYSTEM • EXERCISE • ISOMETRIC EXERCISES • MUSCLE • PHYSICAL FITNESS • REST AND RELAXATION

Q & A

I feel tense all the time. Could yoga help me relax?

Yoga is aimed at relaxing both the body and the mind. The asanas, or postures, are also performed slowly and gracefully, so the mind is soothed while the body is exercised. Breathing exercises and relaxation postures are good for relieving tension.

I'm sure I can't do the difficult postures I see in yoga books. Is that what yoga's about?

No. You have seen postures for advanced students. There is a wide range of simple and graceful exercises for beginners. However, with practice, you will eventually be able to get into postures that you once thought were completely impossible.

My eight-year-old sister wants to take up yoga. Is she too young?

No. Her youthful flexibility will give her a great advantage. The exercises will teach her body control, concentration, gracefulness, and the ability to relax. She will probably progress fast and soon be able to master complicated postures.

Index